MISS
AMBLER'S
Household Book of
GEORGIAN
CURES AND
REMEDIES

MISS
AMBLER'S
Household Book of
GEORGIAN
CURES AND
REMEDIES

MARILYN YURDAN
AND NICOLA LILLIE
ILLUSTRATED BY LAURA LILLIE

The History Press

First published 2013 as *Lavender Water and Snail Syrup*
This paperback edition first published 2023

The History Press
97 St George's Place, Cheltenham,
Gloucestershire GL50 3QB
www.thehistorypress.co.uk

British Library Cataloguing in Publication Data.
A catalogue record for this book is available from the British Library.

ISBN 978 1 80399 357 7

Typesetting and origination by The History Press
Printed and bound in Great Britain by TJ Books Limited, Padstow, Cornwall

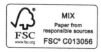

Trees for Life

Contents

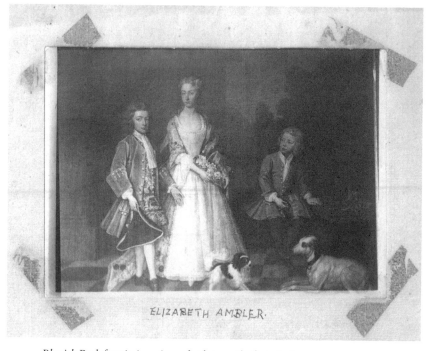

ELIZABETH AMBLER.

Physick Book frontispiece: An early photograph of a painting depicting the Ambler children.

Acknowledgements

Firstly, I would like to thank Marilyn Yurdan for her enthusiasm and work on transcribing the text, and for her writing which illuminates it so well. The multitude of ingredients has been made all the more fascinating by her explanations and details on the historical context.

The Holton Park Archive has been a great inspiration. I would like to extend my thanks to Kevin Heritage and Nigel Phillips for their generosity and the time they have taken to share the archive with me.

I would like to thank Alison Tennant of Tennants Auctioneers, Yorkshire. She has been so helpful since I first discovered that Tennants had sold the three Ambler portraits. I am very grateful to have been allowed to reproduce their photographs of the portraits.

I was delighted to find the watercolour of Spring Grove and am grateful to have been given permission to reproduce it by the City of London, London Metropolitan Archives.

Elisha Biscoe's Free School at Norwood Green is a beautiful building and I want to thank the present owner for her kindness in allowing me to take photographs.

My visit to Spring Grove was wonderful; many thanks to Avril Cutting for her assistance. Thanks also to Annie Hartley for showing me around. At St Leonard's Church, the Archivist, Lawson Cockcroft was very helpful.

Stubbings now has a garden centre in the large walled garden. My thanks go to Dudley and Janine Good for welcoming me and allowing me to photograph the house. Swallowfield is now a collection of apartments. I am grateful to Mrs Philip Jebb for showing me around.

Lastly, I want to thank Laura Lillie for her enthusiasm and commitment to the project. Her prints work well with Marilyn's text as a celebration of Elizabeth Ambler's treasured collection of cures and remedies.

Nicola Lillie
2013

Authors' Note

In his Dictionary of the English Language, published in 1755, Dr Samuel Johnson defines a recipe as 'a medical prescription' and a receipt as a 'prescription of ingredients for any composition'. Usage appears to have inclined towards 'receipt' for medical and 'recipe' for culinary concoctions until the former came only to mean an acknowledgment of something supplied. It should be mentioned that Johnson's doctorates (1765 from Trinity College, Dublin, and 1775 from the University of Oxford) were both honorary ones, and that he held no medical qualifications whatsoever.

Preface

Oxford

In July 1992, I received a parcel from my godmother, Aunt Diana, who lived in Canada. It was just as exciting as her parcels had always been when I was a child – but different. On the Customs declaration form was written: '23 old forks & spoons. 3 ornaments. 1 old recipe book.'

As it transpired, the ornaments were actually a Georgian silver teapot, jug and bowl. These were embellished with the Biscoe family crest depicting a greyhound and hare beneath an oak tree. The forks and spoons bore the same crest and were heavy and beautifully shaped. The old recipe book, with brown suede cover and ninety-eight pages of receipts, was particularly intriguing. Inside the book, pasted to the front page, was a very old black-and-white photograph of a

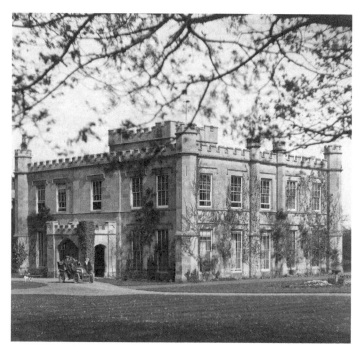

Holton Park, Oxfordshire c.1900. Built by Elizabeth's son Elisha.

portrait. This portrait was of Elizabeth Ambler and her two brothers. Opposite the photograph was the title 'Elizabeth Ambler her Physick Book', and underneath the title had been written at a later date: 'This lady was the 1st wife of Elisha Biscoe & Mother of Elisha Biscoe of Holton Park, Oxford. She died in Bedford Row 11 June 1766 aged 51. She & her husband are buried in the "Vicar's Chancel" at Heston, Middx.' Also added in pencil was 'My great great grandmother.'

At that time, although I loved these objects, I had not realised their significance. I did not understand

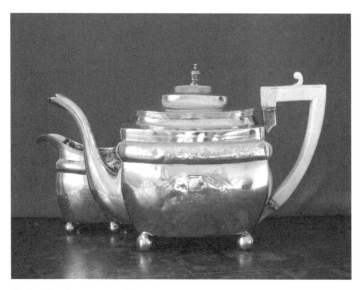

Early Georgian teapot and jug.

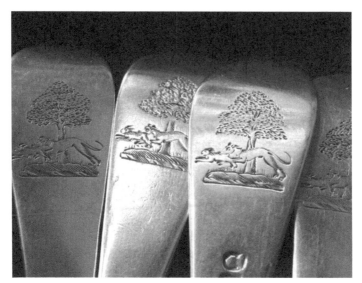

Biscoe crest on Georgian silver forks.

their history, nor did I focus clearly on the period of the eighteenth century, when the Physick Book was compiled. I was busy working, my children were young and I had little time to see that these objects could be a link with the past, a window through which there could be much to discover about my ancestor, Elizabeth Ambler. In 2009, seventeen years later, the silver teapot was in the dresser, polished occasionally, the forks and spoons in the cutlery drawer and the Physick Book set aside in a cupboard. In December that year, whilst visiting Oxford with my son, I had the time to visit Holton Park – a house that was built by Elizabeth's son Elisha Biscoe in 1805. I had visited the house with my mother and grandmother in 1973, when it was a school. Knowing that it had become Wheatley Park School, with many new buildings in the grounds, I had gone to take a quick look at the house but then discovered that a small museum had been created in the old gatehouse. This was a wonderful archive, chronicling the history of the site, including the life of the Tyndale-Biscoe family, descendants of Elizabeth Ambler. The centrepiece of this archive was, for me, a collection of nearly 100 glass photographic plates in wooden boxes, accompanied by a display of the printed photographs. These depicted the Tyndale-Biscoe family and Holton Park and village in the period 1865–1910.

The year 1911 was when the family left Holton, when my grandmother Mollie was 13. Her later life differed considerably from her childhood at Holton

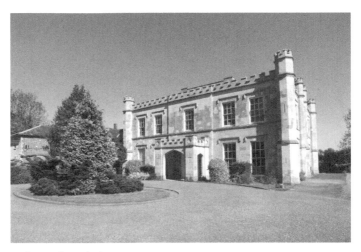

Holton Park, Oxford 2012.

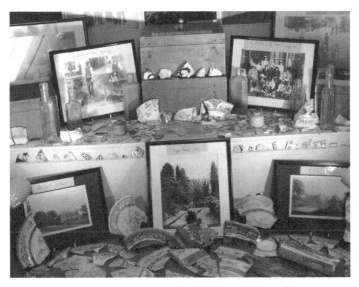

The Holton Park Archive. This particular display includes wooden boxes of glass photographic plates, Tyndale-Biscoe photographs from the 1800s, china and objects found on the Holton Park estate.

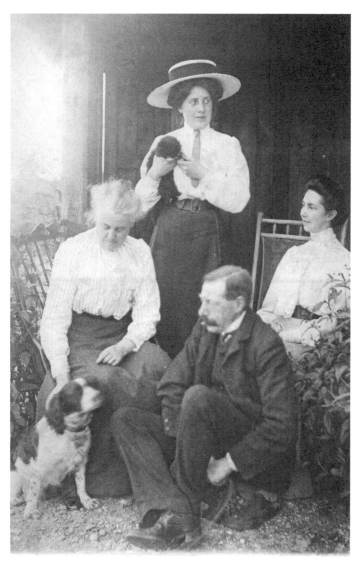

Dorothy Tyndale-Biscoe with her parents Ethel and Stafford, and her Aunt Madge.

and she emigrated to Canada after the Second World War with her two daughters, Diana and my mother Robin, who returned to England to marry my father six months later. My grandmother eventually returned to England but Diana stayed in Canada for the rest of her life, visiting us occasionally, sending lovely parcels and writing regularly. We became quite close, perhaps partly because she had no children herself. Diana had been given a collection of family treasures and history documents by her godmother and aunt, Dorothy. Aunt Dodo, as she was known to

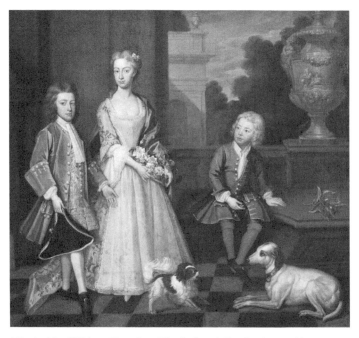

The Ambler Children: Humphry, Elizabeth and Charles. (Painted by Joseph Andre Cellony, 1726)

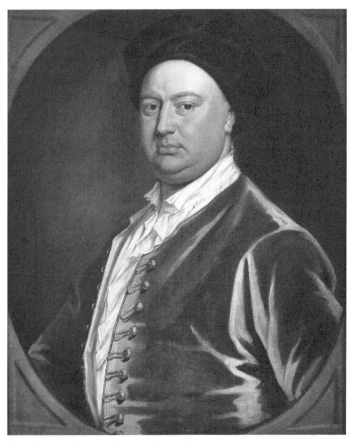

Humphry Ambler. (Attributed to George Knapton)

us, also had no children and was very keen on family history and 'the Family Tree'. She told us many stories when we were young, to which I wish I had listened more carefully. This is how the Physick Book came from Canada to me, I had become the next custodian.

Returning to the archive at Holton and the collection of photographic plates: these belonged to Arthur Tyndale-Biscoe, younger brother of my great-grandfather Stafford. They record the life of the family at Holton and were taken by various members of the family during the period 1865–1910. This visual record of the past, linked not only with the 'Old House' itself but also with great aunts and uncles I had known as a child, was the inspiration for my enthusiasm. The objects and imagery from the past began to take on greater significance and meaning, the more I discovered about the people who owned them. All of this was leading back to Elizabeth Ambler and her Physick Book – fascinating and intriguing to us today, yet a vital part of daily family life to her.

Amongst the photographs at Holton was one of the portrait of Elizabeth and her two brothers, the one that I knew well from the book. This portrait was another focus of my attention and had also been much admired by previous generations, as shown by this excerpt from a memoir by my great uncle Bob, Robert Stafford Tyndale-Biscoe:

… in 1892, after the death of my Grandmother. It was probably at the time of Nata's birth, that one lovely July morning we three children were seated at breakfast with Grandfather. I remember that I was sitting with my back to the windows looking out on the deer park, facing the picture over the fire-place

of our great-great-Grandmother, the lovely Miss
Ambler. Aunt Fanny, who was in charge of the house,
came round and gave each of us a luscious apricot, our
favourite fruit ...[1]

Where was this portrait now? When the house was
sold in 1911 it must have been sold or passed on to
another branch of the family. It was large (2 x 1.75m)
and beautifully painted. Some other Biscoe portraits
went to Jamaica when Robert went to live there,
but this portrait remained in England. While I was
researching online, into other details of the family
history and finding out about Elizabeth's father,
Humphry Ambler, I made a great discovery. Lot 791
from a sale at Tennants Auctioneers appeared on the
screen: a portrait of Humphry Ambler. This was fol-
lowed by a portrait of Anne Breame, his wife. The
annotation read: 'the sitter is the mother of the children in Lot 793.' This was wonderful – Lot 793: the
actual portrait in full colour.

———•••———

---

1   'Tales for Jimmy', Robert Stafford Tyndale-Biscoe, 1962–63.

Elizabeth Ambler and her Family

The portrait of Elizabeth and her two brothers was painted in 1726 when Elizabeth was 14, her brother Humphry was 13 and Charles was 5.

This painting[2] was commissioned by their father Humphry, their mother having died in 1722 when Elizabeth was 10. He was an affectionate and loving father, and in his will he wrote: 'I have an equal and tender love and regard for each of my said children.' He left his fortune to be divided equally between them.

Elizabeth's father was a prosperous lawyer at Middle Temple and the family lived at Bream's Buildings, Chancery Lane. They also lived at Stubbings House, Bisham, Berkshire. This was a mansion house built by Humphry on an 80-acre estate. The land was originally bought as a small portion of oak forest and harvested for sale to shipbuilders.

Humphry and Anne had three other children who died in infancy: Ann, Bream and Amelia. The children's baptisms are all recorded at St Dunstan in the West, Fleet Street. (Humphry also had a daughter Mary, baptised at Bisham in 1719. She may have been the child of Mary Wheatley, a servant at Stubbings, who cared for his children and for him in later life.) Elizabeth's brother Humphry had a fall from a tree

---

2 Painted by Joseph Andre Cellony (1696-1746).

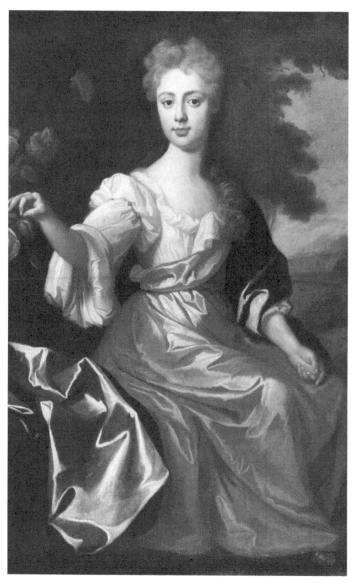

Anne Bream, Mrs Humphry Ambler. (Attributed to Sir Godfrey Knellor)

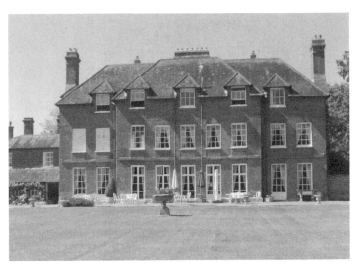

Stubbings: The house built Humphry Ambler near Maidenhead, Berkshire.

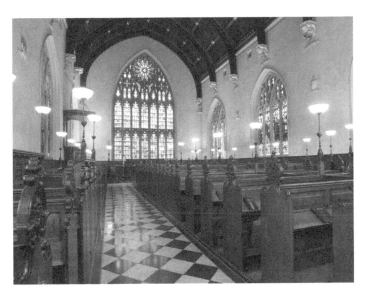

Lincoln's Inn Chapel. Elizabeth and Elisha were married here in 1746.

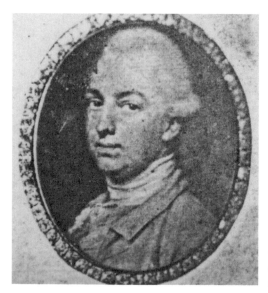

Elisha Biscoe.
Elizabeth's son,
b.1754

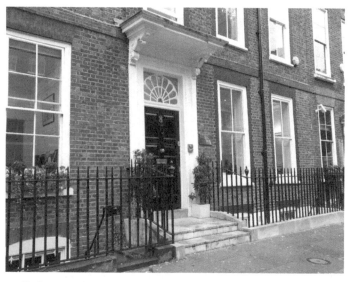

Bedford Row, Holborn, London. Elizabeth and Elisha lived at Bedford Row.
This photograph shows No. 8, which still retains many original features.

while at boarding school at Greenwich, when he was around 8 years old. This resulted in a serious back injury, causing him to suffer from epileptic fits which eventually led to brain damage and an inability to live independently. He died in 1752, aged 39. Her younger brother Charles became a successful lawyer and politician, later becoming attorney to Queen Charlotte. He married Ann Paxton and they had two sons who sadly died while at Harrow School. He and his wife lived at Stubbings and also at Queen Square, Bloomsbury.

Elizabeth married Elisha Biscoe in 1746 at Lincoln's Inn Chapel, one year after her father died. She was 34 at the time of their marriage and she had two children, Anne in 1749 when she was 37 and Elisha in 1754 when she was 42. Her husband was a wealthy lawyer and landowner. He was involved in property development in London, building fifty-six houses and a chapel at Brompton Row, Knightsbridge. He also owned land and property in London, Middlesex, Herefordshire, Buckinghamshire and Oxfordshire. They lived at Bedford Row, Holborn, and also at Spring Grove, Heston, a mansion house that he built in 1754. Elisha was a philanthropist, concerned with helping those most in need. He built and endowed a 'free school' at Norwood in 1767 for poor children in Heston, Hayes and Norwood, providing a sound education and clothing for the pupils. He also bequeathed funds to hospitals, debtors' prisons (the Marshalsea, Newgate and Whitechapel), workhouses and other institutions

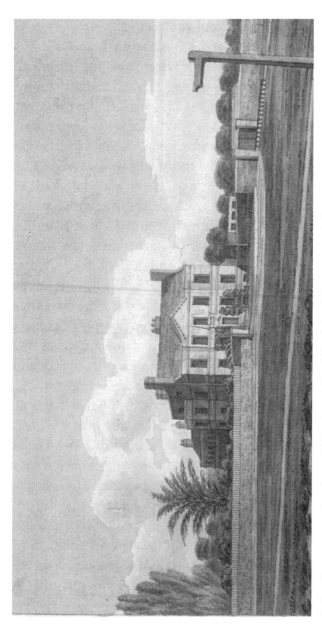

Spring Grove: a watercolour from c.1800 when Sir Joseph Banks lived there, renting the house from the Biscoe family, prior to purchasing the estate in 1808.

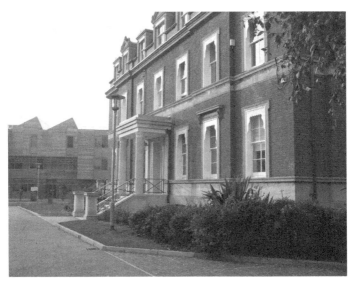

Spring Grove, Heston. The mansion house Elisha Biscoe built in 1754.

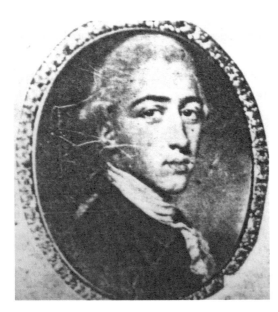

Timothy Hare Earle who married Elizabeth's daughter, Anne.

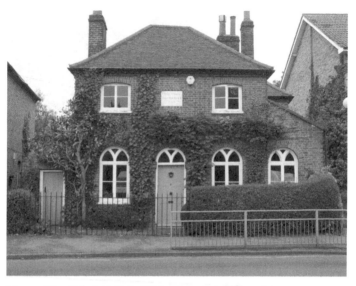

Norwood Free School. Built by Elisha Biscoe in 1767.

in London to provide money, food and clothing for the poor.

Elizabeth must have shared her husband's concerns and aims in life. Sadly, she died in 1766 at the age of 54, having been married for twenty years; thus she did not live to see the results of his philanthropy. Her daughter Anne was 17 and her son Elisha was 12. Their father remarried in 1767 to Frances Western and had a daughter, Catherine, in 1771. Anne and her brother were close and once she was married[3] and their father had died (in 1776) Elisha came to live with the family.

---

3 Married to Timothy Hare Earle in 1772.

Some of the aspects of Elizabeth's life, outlined here, illustrate that life was far from easy for her and her family. Despite having the wealth to reside in beautiful houses with a fair amount of luxury, there was a concern not only for supporting others in the community but also for the difficulties of more immediate family members. For Elizabeth, family life would have involved caring for her epileptic brother and for her ailing father – she only married after he died, relatively late at the age of 34. The Physick Book must certainly have been relied on for remedies and cures, in a more difficult and less certain world. It would also have been passed on down the family for reference and support.

Elizabeth's Descendants and the Physick Book

It seems probable that the book would have been given to Anne after her mother died. Anne and her husband, with their growing family, lived by the Thames at Holme Park, Sonning, Berkshire and at Shiplake Court, then at Swallowfield Park, Berkshire. They 'lived in very grand style' there until 1816.[4] Anne's daughter Mary married Thomas Tyndale in 1808; he was a vicar who took up the living at Holton.[5] In 1819, Anne and her two other daughters, Elizabeth and Letitia, moved to Holton. By then, the Earles' wealth had declined, due to the depreciation of their property in St Kitts, West Indies. Elisha, however, had inherited a great deal from his father and from his uncle, Charles Ambler, enabling him to make Holton the new family home.

Elisha had built a new house at Holton Park in 1805 and this house was eventually inherited by Mary's son, William Earle Tyndale. He married Elizabeth Sandeman and they had a large family of seven boys and one girl.[6] The family name became Tyndale-Biscoe. My great-grandfather Stafford inherited Holton from

---

4 Swallowfield and its Owners' by Lady Constance Russell, 1901.
5 Thomas Tyndale was of the family of William Tyndale, biblical translator and martyr.
6 Henry Stafford, Frances, Albert, Cecil, Edward, Julian, George, Arthur.

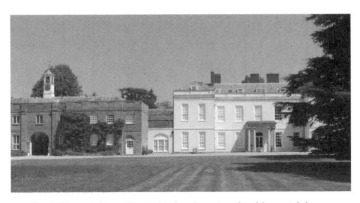

Swallowfield, Berkshire. Elizabeth's daughter Anee lived here with her husband Timothy Hare Earle and their five children.

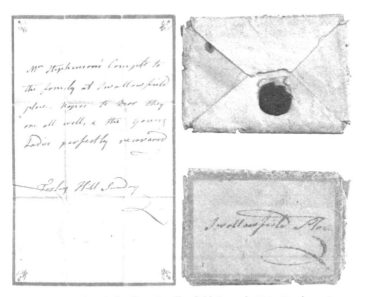

Visiting note to Anne's family at Swallowfield. It reads: "Mrs Stephenson's compliments to the family at Swallowfield Place. Hopes to hear that they are well and perfectly recovered, Farley Hill Sunday."

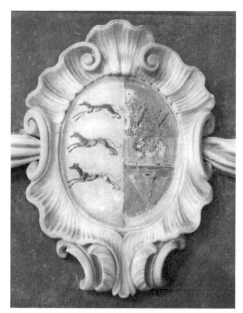

*Biscoe and Ambler crest
on the monument to
Elisha and Elizabeth
in St Leonard's
Church, Heston.*

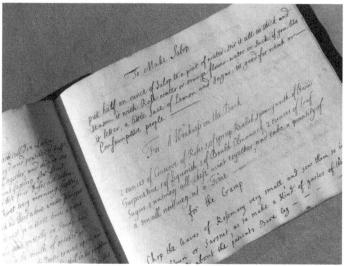

*Physick Book, detail showing receipts written by three different people. Some
were written by Elizabeth, others by family members and friends.*

William and also had a large family with his wife Ethel Frances Primrose.[7] William's family, his children and grandchildren, are the subjects of the photographic plates to be found in the archive collection.

In the family, Letitia, Frances (Fanny) and Dorothy (Dodo) took on the role of chroniclers, writing memoirs and recording interesting facts about the family and the houses where they lived. The Physick Book may have passed down the family thus: Elizabeth – Anne – Letitia – Fanny – Dorothy – Diana – myself. As the book has been inherited through the family, the cures and remedies have naturally been replaced by other medicines and treatments. However, it contains a wealth of information for us today, telling us much about domestic life and health in the eighteenth century. As custodian of the book, I am pleased to have the opportunity of sharing this family treasure.

---

7 Francis, Robert, Archie, Dorothy, Nata, Jack, Tom, Mollie.

Introduction

Medical Care in Elizabeth Ambler's Time

The medical facilities accessible to the Amblers and their neighbours in the eighteenth century were very different from those with which we are familiar today. Apart from the obvious fact that no free state health care was available and the vast difference in levels of technological knowledge, the main difference in patient-practitioner relationships was that the latter were not protected by any form of legislation. Medicine and healthcare was available to anyone who could afford it, in an open market, as the array of advertisements in contemporary newspapers shows.

Another major difference was that hospitals were used only by those who had no family to look after them and were too poor to be treated elsewhere. Not without reason, hospitals were looked on with dread as places full of infection that patients might well not leave alive.

The convenient, and largely theoretical, hierarchy of physicians, surgeons and apothecaries scarcely existed over the country as a whole, although it may have done so in London at some point. At the pinnacle was an elite composed of Oxbridge physicians, the only practitioners permitted to become Fellows of London's Royal College.

Under them came those physicians who had trained elsewhere, many who had excellent practical training acquired at 'foreign' universities such as Leiden, Glasgow and, in particular, Edinburgh. However, wherever they had been trained, physicians did not believe in soiling their hands by actually touching their patients, let alone performing operations on them.

Below these less-exalted physicians came the surgeons, their official body being the Company of Surgeons. Until 1745, its members had been associated with the Barbers' Company. A surgeon's apprenticeship normally served seven years, one or two of which might be spent at a university such as Edinburgh or Glasgow studying a curriculum which included anatomy and chemistry, to which they would not have had access in their home towns. The picture of surgeons as semi-literate blood-letters and bonesetters is inaccurate. The poet John Keats, for

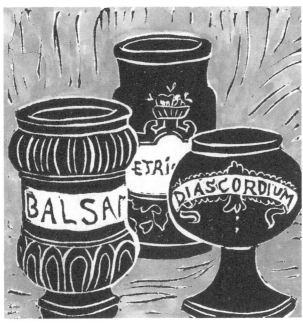

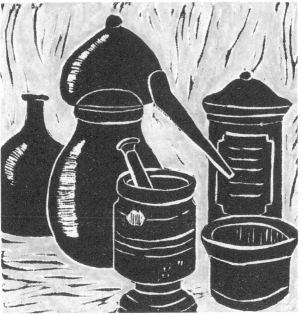

example, spent several years training to be a surgeon, and was also licensed as an apothecary.

Fourthly, and nominally under the supervision of the College of Physicians, came the Society of Apothecaries, formed in 1617 when that body became independent of the Grocers' Company. The function of an apothecary was to dispense as physicians prescribed, although after the Rose Case of 1704, they were themselves permitted to prescribe, providing that they charged only for medicines used and asked for no consultation fee. According to the Apothecaries Act of 1815, the normal qualification for practice as an apothecary would involve the possession of a licence from the Society of Apothecaries (LSA) given after an apprenticeship, taking specified courses, some hospital experience and passing examinations.

Some medical students, including those at St Thomas' Hospital, studied under an apothecary before starting their surgical training. The status of an apothecary was higher than that of the modern chemist as both physicians and surgeons were reliant on his skills in dispensing.

It is debatable whether these bodies were formed in order to protect both members and patients, and to enforce an accepted code of practice, or to establish a monopoly by means of a closed shop; one suspects the latter. By the late eighteenth century, however, the College of Physicians had largely lost the struggle to create this monopoly, and found its self-imposed

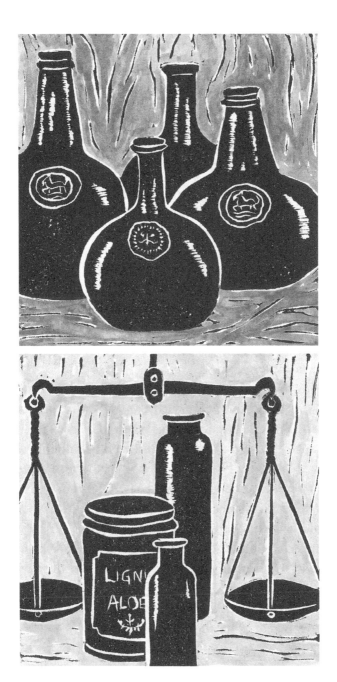

task of controlling surgeons and apothecaries impossible, let alone the ranks of outsiders. The tools of the trade for a surgeon were neither difficult nor expensive to obtain, consisting mainly of bleeding equipment and that for cauterising and cupping. Surgeon-apothecaries, being of similar social background to the majority of patients, were much more welcome than the university-educated physician, as well as being much cheaper to consult.

As the family of a successful lawyer, the Amblers would have been respected members of their communities in the Thames Valley and in London. They would have known physicians socially as they moved in the same circles, as well as consulting them in their professional capacity when they needed a diagnosis or medication prescribed.

However, on an everyday basis they would have had much more contact with the local surgeons and apothecaries. From Stubbings, the most accessible of these would have been in Henley and Maidenhead. Surgeons would be summoned to attend and if necessary operate on patients at the house or on the estate, rather than on their own premises. Elizabeth would visit the shops of the apothecaries of her choice in order to purchase what items she needed for her own store of medicaments, as well as handing over receipts for the apothecary to make up. By coincidence, Elizabeth Ambler's future husband, Elisha Biscoe, had apothecaries in his ancestry.

Patent medicines, for example elixirs and sovereign remedies, as those that came highly recommended for their efficacy were known, were advertised in newspapers and on posters, and could be purchased from nominated agents in towns and cities.

Physick books were by no means unusual and medieval 'leech-books' survive. Many can be found in leading libraries as well as in special collections, such as those at the Wellcome Institute and in the archives of historic houses. Some are written in one or two hands, but others, like Elizabeth's, are the work of a number of people, probably over many years. Elizabeth Ambler's book, however, is most unusual in that it has been in the same family, passed down the female line for about three centuries. We know whereabouts it was housed with each successive owner, and the size and composition of the households that it would have served at any given time.

Elizabeth's book contains over 170 receipts of which the great majority of contributors are named. Among these are: five physicians, Sir Edward Hulse, Doctors Mead, Nisbitt, Saunders and Taylor; ten men who may have been surgeons and/or apothecaries as they are referred to as 'Mr'; fifty-two private individuals; one nurse; four ladies; and two sirs.

Some of the contributions were from the printed works of respected medical men, a few were patent concoctions, but most were collected from family

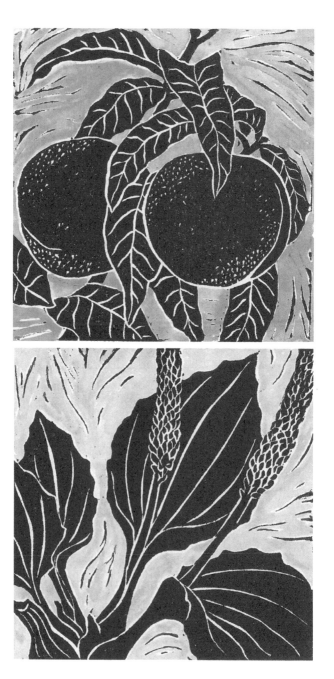

members, friends and neighbours. It would seem that contributors were asked to write their offering themselves rather than dictate them, so that the whole forms a sort of autograph book. The receipts appear in a wide variety of different types of handwriting, ranging from the educated to the barely literate. It has been impossible to ascertain the period over which the book was compiled; however, a few of the receipts appear to date back to well before its start, notably Sir Walter Raleigh's offering on the plague.

It was the responsibility of the lady of the house to act primarily as a dispenser of first aid in the case of accidents, and a supplier of advice and medication for illnesses ranging from indigestion to cancer. Some of the treatments were aimed at prevention, the majority at bringing about a cure, while others were palliative and could only give relief from pain and irritation.

Someone who was intelligent and fully literate was needed to compile and consult physick books and to deal with apothecaries and surgeons when the need arose. While ladies of Elizabeth's social status would appoint and train reliable help in the stillroom, kitchen and herb gardens, they maintained overall control of expensive and potentially lethal ingredients.

Furthermore, they acted as transmitters of folk knowledge of herbs and spices from generation to generation. The ingredients in Elizabeth's book are very typical of this period, when medical receipts were a fascinating combination of something very similar to alchemy, a straightforward use of herbs, spices and chemical compounds that were being introduced. Although there is no mention of spells or other magical activity, had Elizabeth and her peers been poverty-stricken spinsters or widows living in hovels, they may well have been seen as white witches rather than the wives and daughters of respected landowners.

Stubbings, and the other Ambler and Biscoe homes, would have had an extensive kitchen garden and probably a separate herb garden. Much of that which was produced in these gardens was used for both culinary and medicinal purposes. Plants which we now grow only for their flowers, such as roses, carnations and lavender, appear in many receipts, as do others which we consider wild flowers at best and weeds at worst.

The range of herbs, spices, roots and berries imported from abroad is very surprising to the modern eye. The Amblers would have been able to obtain them, at a considerable cost, from contacts who were merchants in the East Indies, and sugar plantation and slave owners in the Caribbean. Obviously, this would have posed no problem in London, but even in provincial Henley apothecaries would have been supplied by boats which then were able to navigate the Thames as far as that town.

As scientific knowledge improved and the chemical industry expanded, the apothecary's work was gradually taken over by that of the pharmacist. However, to this day some 70 per cent of modern medicines are derived from plants and their extracts synthesised to an increasing degree.

Enter the Kitchen:
The Old Recipe Book

Larder Essentials

Dr Mead's Receipt to make Asses' Milk

Take the white of an egg and put a lump
of sugar into it and beat it till the sugar
is dissolved, then put it into half a pint of
red cow's milk and drink it as you do real
asses' milk.

Five of the receipts of Dr Richard Mead (1673–1754) appear in Elizabeth's book. In 1702, Mead had published *A Mechanical Account of Poisons*, the work that made his name in the world of medicine. The following year he was elected physician at St Thomas' Hospital where he helped to persuade Thomas Guy to found the hospital which bears his name, in order to help ease patient pressure on St Thomas' due to the rapid population increase of the capital. In 1703, the young Mead was elected Fellow of the Royal Society; further achievements included lecturing in anatomy at Surgeons' Hall, attending the deathbed of Queen Anne in 1714, and two years later being elected Fellow of the Royal College of Physicians. At the same time he continued to build up a fashionable practice and among his most illustrious patients were Sir Isaac Newton, Sir Robert Walpole (the first prime minister) and the Prince and Princess of Wales. In 1727, he became Physician in Ordinary to George II and Queen Caroline, and his income was rumoured to be a colossal £6,000 a year. Dr Mead was an enthusiastic supporter of inoculating against smallpox and in 1721, sixty years before Edward Jenner's work on vaccination, he took charge of the inoculation of seven condemned criminals at Newgate Prison, all of whom recovered.

Asses' milk: William Buchan MD wrote in his *Domestic Medicine* (Manchester, 1819):

'Asses' milk is commonly reckoned preferable to any other; but it cannot always be obtained … I have known very extraordinary effects from asses' milk in obstinate coughs, which threatened a consumption of the lungs; and do verily believe, if used at this period, that it would seldom fail … If the milk should happen to purge, it may be mixed with old conserve of roses. When that cannot be obtained, the powder of crabs' claws may be used in its stead. When a cough, a difficulty of breathing, or other symptoms of a consumption, succeed to the small-pox, the patient must be sent to a place where the air is good, and put upon a course of asses' milk, with such exercise as he can bear.'

Apricock Ratifia

Take a Gallon of the best Brandy,
300 apricocks, almonds two dozen and a
half apricocks, divide them, take 3 quarters
of a pound of white sugar candy broken in
lumps, 9 fine Newington peaches, 3 fine
nectarines and cut them in pieces. Put all
these into a glass jar, lett it stand a fortnight then stir them every fortnight, and at
two months end it is made. Note: strain it
out and let it stand a month and then strain
it again and do so until it is fine.

Apricock: not a misspelling or the result of someone
hearing the word 'apricot' incorrectly. 'Apricock'
derives from the Latin *praecox*, meaning early, in
this case early ripening.

Ratafia: an alcoholic drink flavoured with the ker-
nels of cherries, peaches or other fruit, as well as
apricots, spiced, and sweetened with sugar.

A gallon: 8 pints or 4.55 litres.

Newington peaches: a variety of peach thought to
have been so named because they were first
grown at Newington Butts in South London.

To Make Ginger Bread

One pound of flour, six ounces of butter,
six ounces of coarse sugar and one ounce
of dried ginger powdered up in an ounce
of Jamaica pepper, one ounce of caraway
seeds. Mix the butter with the flour as fine
as possible and put in an ounce of treacle
(if wanted) [and] a spoonful of water that
has been boiled and stood to be cold, then
mix all these ingredients together and put
in a slack oven.

Jamaica pepper: *Pimenta officinalis*, the more usual
name of which is allspice.
A slack oven: one that burns slowly.

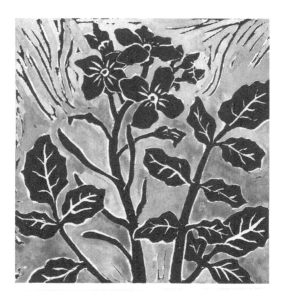

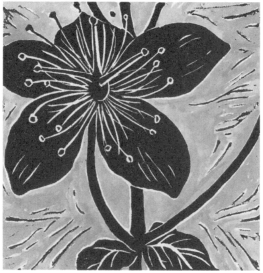

To Make Lavender Water

Strip the lavender from off the stalks and
fill the pot for the alembic almost full
with them, then put to them about three
quarts of cider and draw off two quarts.
If you would have it very fine, then you
must take the same quantity of flowers
and put to it one quart of cider and two
quarts of water and drain it off as before,
but take care that it don't burn nor boil
too fast.

A Quart: 2 pints

Mrs Davison's Receipt for Snail Milk Water

Take four quarts of new milk, two quarts of sack carduus, ground ivy, balm, of each one handful. Sixty ox-eye daisies, one handful of millipedes, fifty shell snails, well purged with fennel, sixty earth-worms slit and an ounce and a half of balsam of Tolu. Still all in a cold still; drain off four quarts. Drink a quarter of a pint going to bed, at eleven in the morning and at five in the afternoon or at any time when thirsty. This receipt is for a grown up person and must be given in proportion for a child.

Millipedes: or woodlice, are frequently found in seventeenth-century receipts but their use was largely discontinued in the eighteenth century, suggesting that this is one of the older receipts in Elizabeth Ambler's collection.

Balsam of Tolu: this balsam takes its name from a town in Colombia, now named Santiago de Tolu. It is produced from the resin of *Myroxylon balsamum* (formerly *M. toliuferum*)

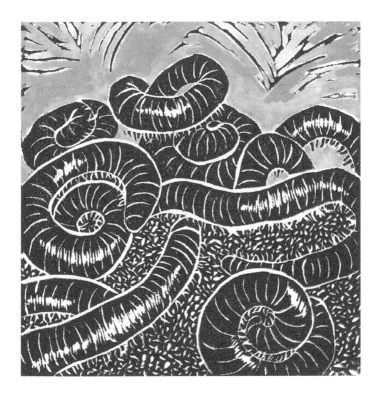

which is collected and allowed to harden in
the sun.

Sack carduus: white Spanish wine in which the
carduus thistle has been steeped.

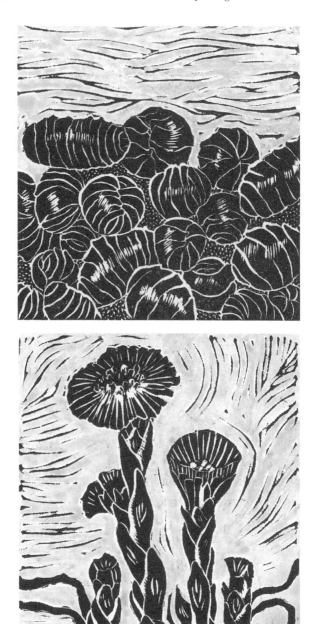

Snaile Water

One peck of garden snails, two pecks of
ground ivy, two gallons of spring water,
one gallon of milk: ingredients to be distilled in a cold still, a quart to be taken
the first thing in the morning and the
same quantity going to bed, sweetened
with capulaire.

Capulaire: capillaire, a type of syrup made from
maidenhair fern in syrup flavoured with orange
blossom or orange-blossom water.

Syrup of Snails

Take shell snails when the dew is upon
them, take their shells off and slit them.
To one pound of snails put half a pound
of white sugar candy fairly powdered; put
half to the slit snails in a flannel bag, the
other half of the sugar into an earthen
basin. Hang your bag over the basin for
your snails to drop into it. Set in a cellar or
damp place to melt the sugar candy.

Lady Chesterfield's Receipt to make Whay [Whey]

Put in the evening three pints of milk
(if poor) or one quart (if rich) into a flat
earthen pan and next morning skim off
the cream entirely; put the milk into a
well-seasoned earthen pipkin that holds
two or three quarts or five pints. Let it boil
on a gentle heat. When it boils up to the
top put in one dram of Cream of Tartar.
Take it off the fire, let it boil up a second
time then put in another dram of Cream
of Tartar, let it boil a little then take it off
the fire, cover the pipkin and let it stand
by the fire for about half an hour, then
pour it into a basin and drink it.

Cream of Tartar: the common name for potassium
hydrogen tartrate, which is obtained from the
sediment produced in the wine-making process.
Pipkin: a small earthenware pot used for boiling.

Mrs Shank's Receipt to make Vipers Broth

Take a small chicken, skin it, boil it six
minutes in a quart of water then put the
viper in and boil it four minutes, then
strain it off. Let the patient take a quarter
of a pint, three times a day.

Viper broth: thought to be both nourishing and
invigorating. The peak of its popularity was in
the early eighteenth century.

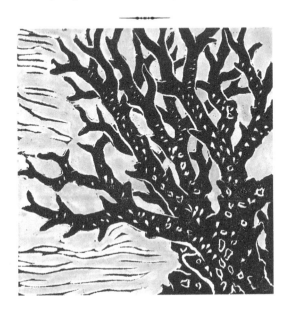

The Famous Water called Dr Stevens's Water

Take a gallon of French wine, cloves, mace, caraway, coriander, fennel seeds, gallinga, ginger, cinnamon grains, nutmeg, niseed each a dram, to these add camomile, sage, mint, rue, red rose, pellitory, the roots of fennel, parsley and setwall, of each 4 ounces and having bruised them, put them into two quarts of Canary and the like quantity of ale, and then having stood sixteen hours with often stirring, draw off the quintessence by Alembic over a soft fire.

Gallinga: galangal.

Setwall: a variety of valerian.

Canary: a fortified wine from Spain or the Canary Islands.

An Alembic: a piece of apparatus used in the distilling process. Often shown in pictures of alchemists, it was the forerunner of the modern retort.

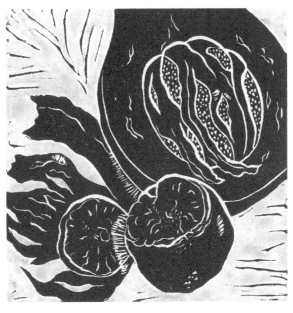

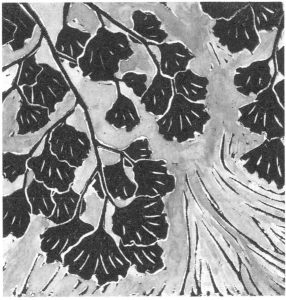

Fevers and Diseases

Mrs Robinson's Receipt for Ague

Take the snuff of a candle, add to it an
equal quantity of nutmeg, grated, and
half an hour before the fit is expected give
it to the patient in a glass of warm water
and white wine. If 'tis a child, the powder
must be about as much as will lay upon a
sixpence, and a grown person as will lay
upon a shilling. You must lay the snuff
of candle upon a piece of white paper to
dry then pound it and mix it with your
nutmeg. This receipt all ways stops the
third fit and often prevents the second
fit coming; has never been known to fail
of a case. The patient must go to bed as
soon as they have taken the medicine for it
causes great perspiration.

Ague: (pronounced 'ayg-yoo') a malarial infection
marked by chills, fever and sweating which
recur at regular intervals. Depending on length
of time between attacks, the different types
were known as the quotidian or daily ague, the
tertian which returned every second day, the
quartan which returned every third day, and

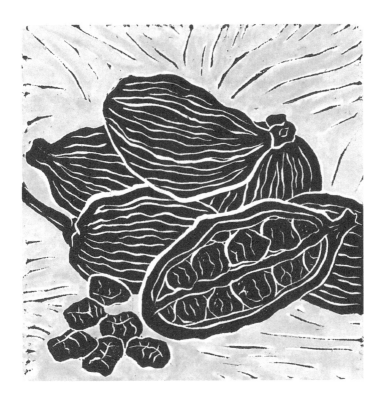

the quintan every fourth day. Johnson notes,
'An intermittent fever, with cold fits succeeded
by hot.'

Ague fit: the paroxysm of the ague.

Snuff: a candle's burnt wick.

To Make a Red Powder for
a Feaver 'our own way'

Take a quart of white wine and half a spoonfull
of Rose water, wormwood, mugwort, carduus
dragon, southernwood, chamomile, scabuis [sca-
bious], snackell, betony, hartshorn, wild sage,
thyme, burdock roots, lovage, thistle, celandine,
wall-flower leaves, feverfew, of each a small,
and red nettles, brookline, bay leaves, single
heartsease, mint, pennyroyal, tamarisk, borage,
angelica finger, dock, of each a small handful. Cut
them small and steep them in the wine 24 hours.
Take a pound of the best bole armonack, then
take your wine, as much as will make it as soft as
pap. Sett it in the sun in a basin, stirring it once
or twice a day. When it begins to grow thick and
dry, add more of the wine to it and continue till
[as] you began. Then take metridate, London
Treacle Diascordium, alhermes, black crabs' claws
finely beaten, of each 2 ounces, 2 drachms of
snake root finely powdered, bezoar, ambergris,
red coral, white amber, of each 2 drams. Stir these
together in the sun till they be dry and come to
the thickness of a plaister, then make them up in
little balls or cakes as you please, then dry them
for your use; 'they must be maid in May.'

Carduus: a type of thistle, most commonly the blessed, holy or milk thistle.

Snackell: snake oil, now used as a general term for a quack cure-all. Real snakes were used medicinally (see Viper Broth), and Egyptian dried vipers were considered very desirable.

Brookline: *Veronica beccabunga*, a plant related to speedwell, which was eaten in salads and often found with and eaten with watercress, with which it is also used medicinally. Alternative spellings are 'brooklime' or 'brook lime' and another name is 'water-pimpernel'.

Bole armonack: *Bole armoniac*, an astringent, clay-like earth.

Metridate: an expensive medicine taken as an electuary and containing many ingredients. It was considered to be a remedy against all manner of poisons and infections. The name comes from King Mithridates who, according to legend, made himself immune to poisons by regularly taking them in tiny doses as antidotes.

Diascordium: a medicine made from dried herbs, especially *Teucrium scordium*, the water germander, but over the years the ingredients varied considerably. Among other complaints, it was used for plague and syphilis.

Alhermes: a liquid coloured by kermes, the bodies of female insects, *Coccus ilicis*, which yield a reddish-coloured dye.

Bezoar: a stone-like concretion found in the stomachs or intestines of certain ruminant animals, especially the wild goat of Persia. It was supposed to have medicinal qualities.

Plaister: an older spelling of plaster.

Receipt against the Plague

Take of rue, mint, rosemary, wormwood and lavender a handfull of each, infuse them together in a gallon of white wine vinegar; put the whole into a stone pot, closely covered up and pasted over the cover. Sett the pot thus closed, upon warm wood ashes for eight days, after which draw off (or strain through fine flannell) the liquid and put it into bottles, well cork'd, and into every quart bottle put a quarter of an ounce of camphor. With this preparation wash your mouth and rub your loins and your temples every day. Snuff a little up your nostrils when you go into the air, and carry about with you a bit of sponge dipped in the same, in order to smell to upon all occasions, especially when you are near any place or person that is infected.

Any body inclined to a Consumpsion, Mrs Steaven's Receipt

Drink every morning red cow's milk upon
balm and pennyroyal and sweetened with
conserve of roses or ginger root.
3 pints or 2 quarts of candid water,
5 ounces of hartshorn, 1 ounce of candid
ginger root, 1 ounce of caraway comforts
and 4 pipings of nutmeg.
A pint of milk, 3 spoonfulls of red roses'
water, 5 spoonfulls of planting water,
1 ounce of sugar of roses.

Consumption: an old word for pulmonary tuberculosis, it was later superseded by the word 'phthisis'. Johnson described consumption thus:

'In physick, a waste of muscular flesh. It is frequently attended by a hectick fever [one which accompanies consumption and similar diseases and is marked by flushes] and is divided by physicians into several kinds, according to the variety of its causes.'

Hartshorn: shavings from deer antler used as gelatine.
Pipings of nutmeg: water in which nutmeg has been boiled.

Mrs Sweet's Excellent Receipt for a Consumption or a Cough

Take a pint of oil of turpentine, 4 ounces of flower of brimstone, an ounce and a half of letharges of gold.
Let them be prepared in a sand heat.
Take seven drops on a moist spoonful of sugar morning and evening for three days and rest three days then take nine drops morning and evening [for] three days then rest three days again. Eat no cheese and leave off other medicines.

Brimstone: a common name for sulphur.
Letharges: the left-over scum or ashes after boiling or burning.
Sand heat: heated sand in which a vessel was placed to give an even temperature.

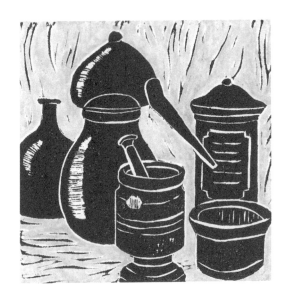

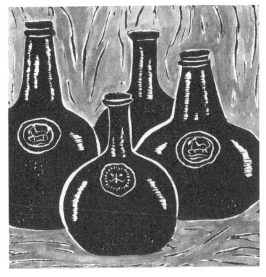

Sir Walter Rawleigh's Receipt against Plague

Take three pints of Malmsey or Canary sack, boyle in it one handful of sage and as much rue, till one pint is wasted away, then strain it and set it over the fire again and put thereto one dram of long pepper, half an ounce of ginger and a quarter of an ounce of nutmeg, all well beaten together. The let it boil a little and put thereto one dram and half of methridate, one dram of Venice Treacle and a quarter of a pint of aqua vitae or hot angelica water.

Keep this as your life above all worldly treasures; take it always morn and eve, three spoonfuls at a time if the party be disease[d], if not, every morn is sufficient in all the plague time trust to this, for certainly God be praised, for it, there was never man, woman or child whom this drink deceived, if the heart was not poisoned or drowned with the disease before.

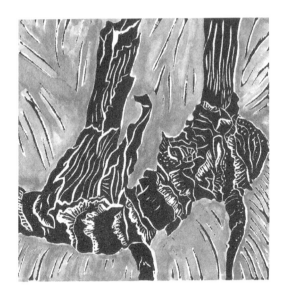

Malmsey and Canary: general names for fortified wines from Spain or the Canary Islands.

Long pepper: *Piper longum*, which looks a little like a catkin, is good for throat irritations and, it is claimed, leads to long life.

Venice treacle: an electuary on a honey (later molasses) base, particularly useful against venom, but with many other properties. First developed in Italy, it was later exported from Venice throughout Europe, hence its name.

Methridate: see note on p. 65.

Wounds

To make an Unparalleled Balsam, Mrs Powell's Receipt

Take Balsam of Peru, one ounce Best storax two ounces, Benjamin impregnated with sweet almonds three ounces, aloes succotrina, myrrh, elect. purest frankincense, roots of angelica flowers, of St John's wort, of each half an ounce. Beat these drugs, the balsam excepted, as small as may be. Put them into a bottle then pour on them the Peruvian balsam and one pint of the spirits of wine, then stop the bottle very closely. Set it for 20 or 30 days in the sun during the heat of the summer shake frequently.

The bottle of the balsam will, [at] the end of that time, be fit for use. Let it always remain in the grounds or faeces and when you have occasion to use any of it, pour some into a small bottle and stop it well after you have used it. This excellent medicine may be as well farmed by sand heat, know[n] well to the Apothecary, or in a hot dunghill.

Wound Water

Take equal quantities of Venice turpentine
and highest rectified spirits of wine, but
rather most turpentine of the two. Put
them in a large vial and shake it till it is
perfectly mixed and looks clear. Apply
it to the wound with a feather and as it
dries, wet it again.

Venice turpentine: common turpentine consisted of
oleo resins that are given out by many types of
conifers, the most important of these being the
Mediterranean cluster pine, *Pinus pinaster*, grown
in Les Landes. Venice turpentine was the name
given to that obtained from larch trees in the
Tirol and presumably exported through Venice.

Mrs Randolph's Receipt to make Arqubucade Water: its Virtues are to stop Bleeding if Inward Wound

Take:

Small sage 4 handfuls

Vervine 2 handfuls

Great confire 4

St John's wort 2

Mugwort 4

Wormwood 2

Bugle 2

Fenagle 2

Sinorgle 2

Water bettony 2

Great dary 2

Little dary 2

Long plantin 2

Green tabaco leaves 2

Round plantin 2

Bethony 2

Adgromony 2

Pick all these herbs clean and cut them, put them into an earthen pot and put to them six quarts of the best white wine. Let them steep 24 hours then still it of[f], set the Bottles in the sun six weeks but take them in every night. It will keep many years; drink it, if inner, three times a day a little warm, if outwards wash with it, dip a [piece of] lint in it and lay upon it [i.e. the wound]; it has been given with great success on vomiting.

This receipt follows the modern presentation of listing all the ingredients and the quantities needed in each before giving the method, rather than leaving the reader to sort through the whole receipt to find them.

———•••———

Arquebusade: a type of distilled water made from a range of aromatic plants as in the above recipe. It was originally used to cleanse gunshot wounds and help them to heal.

Confire: (comfrey) *Symphytum officinale* produces a chemical compound called allantoin, which is useful for minor cuts and grazes, also speeds up the healing process in wounds, strains, sprains and broken bones. One of its popular names is knitbone.

Mugwort: *Artemisia vulgaris*, which has antibacterial properties, is popular in the treatment of female disorders and is used to stimulate the uterus in order to bring on delayed menstruation and restore regular periods. Like other bitter herbs, it is excellent for digestive disorders and eases bloating and wind.

Bugle: *Ajuga reptans* is an astringent, analgesic wound healer which is also mildly laxative and a mild liver cleanser.

Sinorgle: this could be *Acacia senegal*, the stem of which yields gum arabic. This forms a soothing, protective coating on inflamed parts of the respiratory, alimentary and urinary tracts. When used with certain astringents, it is prescribed for coughs, sore throats and catarrh, as well as for some types of diarrhoea and dysentery.

Great dary: this is possibly a miscopying of clary, any of the various aromatic herbs of the salvia or sage family. Today clary refers specifically to *Salvia sclarea* which is used to make an eye lotion, a gargle and as an antiseptic.

Long (leaved) plantin: *Plantago lanceolata* or rib-wort. A poultice applied to any skin ailment will work quickly. Plantain leaves can be put on to cuts to stop bleeding.

Round (leaved) plantin: *Plantago major* or common plantain. The various members of the plantain family have similar medicinal properties.

Bethony: (betony) *Betonica officinalis* or *Stachys officinalis* is commonly called woundwort from its use in the treatment of sores and ulcers. At one time it was looked on as a holy herb which would keep away bad dreams and visions and deter devils. Today it is used in the treatment of nervous complaints brought on by stress and anxiety, and to ease headaches and neuralgia caused by stress.

Adgromony: (agrimony) *Agrimonia eupatoria*, also called Aaron's rod and liverwort. Thanks to astringent properties, this plant is effec-tive against diarrhoea, especially in children. Agrimony stops irritation of the urinary tract and so may be useful in treating urinary incontinence, bed-wetting and adult incontinence. However, it was traditionally used in the Middle Ages for staunching the blood from wounds sustained on battlefields. Today it is mainly used as a mild astringent and tonic as the tannins which it contains invigorate the mucus membranes, easing the symptoms of coughs, bronchitis and asthma.

Vervine: (vervain) *Verbena officinalis* is used to relieve the pain caused by many complaints and as a tranquiliser, as an expectorant to treat chronic bronchitis, and to relieve joint pain caused by rheumatism. Modern herbalists use vervain to combat depression brought on by chronic illness. It can also help to heal liver damage.

Wormwood: *Artemisia cina*, or santonica, was used to get rid of internal worms. Its dried flower heads were used for the same purpose.

Fenagle: (fenugreek) *Trigonella foenum-graecum* lowers the level of sugar in the blood. Methi, the bitter seeds of the fenugreek, are used in Indian cuisine and its leaves are used in teas. Because the powerful antioxidants it contains benefit the liver and pancreas, fenugreek is used to treat diabetes and digestive problems as well as to lower cholesterol levels.

The Virtues of the Balsam

It cures all manner of green wounds in 8 or 9 days by dropping it into the wound or applying it with a feather. It will at first cause much pain. Upon applying any other medicine to a wound, a digestion follows, but upon the application of this, none will happen unless there has been an application of some other medicine before and if there has, wash it clean with warm white wine or any other fluid which will cleanse well the wound and then apply as above the balsam, while brown paper dipped in the balsam is a good cover for the wound that has been dressed in it.

Secondly, it cures all contusions, scalds, and burnings, being applied as above and advised to be covered. It is good in all cancerous and scrofulous cases, but then 20 or 30 drops must be inwardly taken in a glass of white wine or any other proper liquor. It cures St Anthony's fire and all manner of boil externally and internally taken as above but then the person should take a little purging physick.

It cures the biting of a mad dog taken in the same manner and any venomous creature, taken in time. Any person that is seized by the smallpox may take it in a little claret, from 5 to 20 or 30 drops, regards being had to their age, every 24 hours till the pox be turned; applying it with a feather will effectually prevent pitting.

It is very good for sore eyes by dropping it into them; by dropping some on lint and applying it to your tooth, ear or in your nostril cures the tooth, ear or head ache effectually.

It cures the colic or any pain in the stomach by taking 20, 30 or 40 drops in any liquor. The internal application of this balsam in any proper vehicle is in great the use in the treatment of a spotted fever, the number of drops being proportioned to the person's age and repeated as often as occasion requires. In all instances above, whether bruises inwardly or outwardly, suffer a due proportion of this balsam to be applied [it] will answer as in human race.

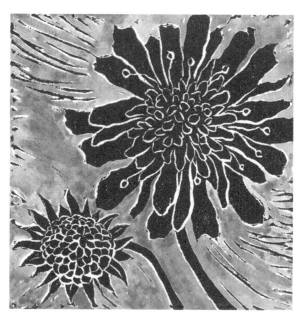

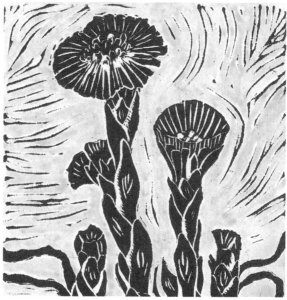

Balsam: is a general term for several types of aromatic resin obtained from trees and shrubs and used as a base for certain medicinal preparations and fragrances. The meaning was also extended to include oily or resinous preparations (which frequently made use of turpentine) in which substances could be dissolved or combined.

Balsam of Peru: the principal use for this balsam today is in aromatherapy and perfumery because of the scent, which is similar to vanilla and cinnamon. However, this resinous oil has antiseptic qualities which assist skin to heal as well as properties common to all balsams. Peruvian balsams were traditionally used to make cough syrups and destroy parasites.

Storax: full name Levant or liquid storax, it is a rare fragrant gum resin which is obtained from a tree, *Styrax officinalis*, grown in the eastern Mediterranean. It was used in medicine as a relaxant as well as in perfumery and making candles and incense.

Benjamin: *Artemisia abrotanum* has the more common names of southernwood and lad's love. Its uses include the treatment of various menstrual problems and its leaves mixed with treacle were used to dispel threadworms in children.

Aloes succotrina: *Aloe succotrina*, comes from South Africa and is a slow-working laxative and astringent as well as having several other uses in the making of pills and medicines.

Elect (electuary of) purest frankincense: an electuary is a medicinal substance mixed with honey or treacle to make it more palatable.

Frankincense: an aromatic gum obtained from trees of the genus Boswellia. Its name means pure incense.

Contusions: another name for bruises.

Cancerous: Johnson defined a cancer as, 'A virulent swelling or sore, not to be cured'.

Scrofulous: relates to scrofula, a type of tuberculosis which leads to swellings in the neck. It was usually found in children and could be caught from drinking unpasteurised milk, although it was usually caused by poor hygiene. Scrofula takes its name from the Latin for sow as the swellings were thought to look like little pigs. Samuel Johnson, who suffered from the disease as a child, called it 'A scrofulous distemper, in which the glands are ulcerated, commonly believed to be cured by the touch of a king'. Johnson was touched for scrofula by Queen Anne, the last monarch to perform this service, on 30 March 1712. However, the royal touch failed to cure him and an operation was performed that left him permanently scarred.

St Anthony's fire: the popular name for erysipelas, so named from the fiery red colour of the areas of affected skin.

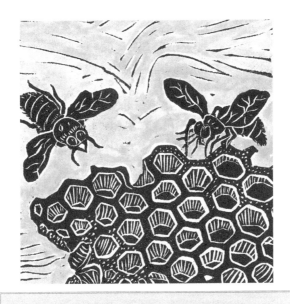

To Heale an old Sore

Take beas wax one ounce, cutt it thine
and melt it down half way then take it of
and stor it till melted, then Cras it ne a
heat and put in 3 ounces of butter from
the Chrum and stor it till melted then put
in Salted In of naturall balsam half the
3 ounces stir all well togeather pott it off
use and work sum in Lint for rents bige
nofe to make rents to fill ofe the orrafis
and as heale make them less and less till
hole Cour the ounce with balsam as before
till well.

Dr Mead's Cure for the Bite of a Mad Dog

Let the patient be blooded at the Arm
nine or ten ounces. Take of the herb
call'd in Latin lichen cinerius terrestris, in
English ash-coloured liverwort, cleaned,
dried and powder'd half an ounce. Of
black pepper powdered two drachms,
mix these well together and divide the
powder into four doses, one of which must
be taken every morning, fasting, for four
mornings successively in half a pint of
cow's milk, warm. After these four doses
are taken, the patient must go into the
Cold Bath or a cold spring or river, every
morning fasting, for a month. He must be
dipt all over but not stay in (with his Head
above water) longer than half a minute, if
the water is very cold. After this he must
go in three times a week for a fortnight
longer. The lichen is a very common herb
and grows generally in sandy and barren
soils all over England. The right time

to gather it is in the month of October or November. I took the liberty, having some acquaintance with the Doctor, to wait upon and discourse with him about this matter as this gentleman is not more distinguished by his skill in his profession than he is by his humanity, he was pleased to tell me that it was not only a powder which he used in this case which in the experience of above 30 years in more than 500 patients, he had never known to fail in success. He said that the sooner the medicine was taken after the bite, the better, though he had often found it to answer tho' not taken till a fortnight or later after it, he added that he never made a secret of this but communicated it to everybody as occasion afford, having indeed mentioned something of it long since in his book of poisons. He very readily gave me his method in writing with leave to make it as publick as I would, and it was the above mentioned. I am your humble servant, Philanthropos.

Fasting: on an empty stomach. Today we still use the term in fasting blood tests.

Blooded at the arm, nine or ten ounces: refers to a practice used by medical men from ancient times until well into the nineteenth century. A small amount of blood was taken from one of the principal veins in order to prevent or cure an amazing range of illnesses, thought to be caused by an imbalance of humours or the blood being too 'rich'. This operation was performed by a barber-surgeon using small, sharp, lancet-like blade called a fleam and the results collected in a bowl kept for the purpose. Other methods of drawing blood were by scarifying the skin with small, razor-like blades and by the application of leeches.

Digestion

To Make an Opening Drink

Liverwort, maiden hair, colt's foot, scabious and unset hyssop, each an handful,
2 ounces of French barley and 4 ounces of
raisins of the sun. These mix with a gallon
of spring water. Let them be boiled till
they become 3 quarts but when they are
all most boiled add a handfull of wood
sorrel and 2 ounces of liquorish.

Opening Drink: one to open the bowels and
cure constipation.

Scabious: field scabious, *Knautia arvensis*, used for
skin troubles and against the plague.

Raisins of the sun: sun-dried grapes, as opposed to
currants which take their name from Corinth
in Greece.

Liquorish: extracted from the root of the plant
Glycyrrhiza glabra; it was used as a medicine
before it was used for confectionery.

To make Stoughton's Elixir, good for a Bad Appetite

Pare off the rinds of six Seville oranges,
very thin, and put them in a quart bottle
with an ounce of gentian, scraped and
sliced and six pennyworth of Cochineal.
Put to it a pint of best brandy, shake it
together two or three times the first day
and then let it stand to settle two days and
clear it off into a bottle for use.
Take a large teaspoonful in a glass of wine in
the morning and at four of the clock in the
afternoon, or you may take it in a dish of tea.

Elixir: a liquid which contains a drug with syrup,
glycerine or alcohol added in order to hide its
unpleasant taste, although traditional practitioners argue that this bitterness stimulates
the blow of bile which aids digestion. This particular recipe was first put together towards
the end of the seventeenth century by Richard
Stoughton, a British apothecary, and was pat-
ented in 1712. His 'elixir' became extremely
popular and was imitated in homes all over the
country. Syrup is made by pouring a pint of
water on to 2lb sugar, heating it until the sugar

dissolves, stirring it all the time until it boils and then removing it from the heat.

Gentian root: *Gentiana lutea* is a bitter herb which will increase gastric secretions and aid the digestive processes. Gentian is also used for gastro-intestinal inflammation of the stomach and intestines.

Cochineal: a bright-red dye obtained from dried and powdered bodies of *Coccus cacti*, insects which live on Central American cacti. Before cochineal was discovered by Europeans sandalwood, known as 'sanders' or 'saunders', was used in cookery. The reference to a dish of tea is a reminder that tea was initially drunk out of dishes or bowls rather than from cups.

Lady Worden's Receipt for the Wind

Take of the powders of liquorish, caraway seeds, fennel seeds and sugar candy finely crushed, of each an ounce, of the powders of rhubarb, cream of tartar of each half an ounce. Mix them together and carry them in a box in your pocket and take three or four times a day, as much at a time as will lie on a sixpence. It generally purges, cools the blood and expels the wind.

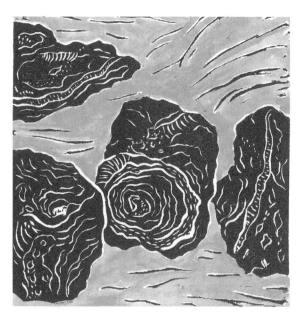

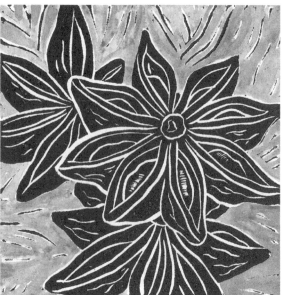

Lady Clark's Receipt to make Glister for the Worms

Take some milk and turn it with treacle
and then strain it and boil in it half an
ounce of worm seeds, bruised, boil it
a little then strain it out and give it as
a glister. This must be often repeated
and is, I believe, one of the best things
in the world. If for grown persons (as
many has worms) it must be an ounce of
worm seeds.
For a child of three years old, try a quarter
of an ounce or less of the worm seeds at
first to see if it agrees.

Worm seeds: those of the plants santonica, or
wormwood.

Mrs Miller's Receipt to make Bitters

Gentian, galangal, zedoary, snake root, of each a dram rhubarb, two drams, saffron, cochineal, each half a dram camomile flowers, half a handfull:
To be infused in a quart of white wine and take[n] 3 or 4 spoonfulls twice a day about eleven in the forenoon and about five or six in the evening. If you please, you may put in a little orange peel and it will make the bitters a good deal better.

Bitters: a type of alcoholic liquor flavoured with bitter herbs and roots which is taken to improve digestion and appetite or cure intestinal worms.

Galangal: the roots of this plant, *Alpinia officinarum*, taste rather like ginger. They were imported from Java and much used as a spice in European cookery. They went out of fashion when replaced by ginger, but have made a return with the growing popularity of Thai cuisine. In medicine it is valued for the treatment of spasms or convulsions as well as in cases of indigestion and lack of appetite.

Zedoary: *Curcuma zedoaria*, a plant found in India and Indonesia related to turmeric which has an

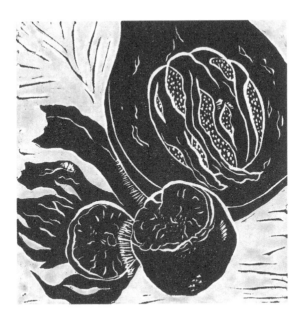

aromatic rhizome. As well as for medicinal purposes, it was used in dyeing and perfumery. In
the West, it has been replaced by ginger.

Snake root: Bistort, or *Polygonum bistorta*, which is
a relative of the sunflower, a plant also related
to turmeric. Its name comes from its use as an
antidote for snake bites.

Dram: in this case an apothecary's drachm which
was one-eighth of an ounce or sixty grains, or as
a fluid measure one-eighth of a fluid ounce.

Boyle's Receipt to strengthen the Bowells

Stick liquorish sliced, a pound of raisins stoned; pour two quarts of barley water scalding hot upon them, cover it till cold then drink it at meals. If you are feverish, then take ten drops of spirits of nitre morning and night in some of the liquor.

Barley water: Aqua hordeata, made by boiling pearl barley in water and used to sooth by forming a protective layer over irritated areas. It was commonly prescribed for by medical men and usually made at home. Its taste was sometimes improved by the addition of lemon or orange juice, making it the forerunner of today's commercial squashes.

Spirits of nitre: a pale yellow liquid with a rather sweet taste and pleasing smell. It is obtained by distilling alcohol with nitric and sulphuric acids, and consists essentially of ethyl nitrite with a small amount of acetic aldehyde. It is used as to induce sweating, encourage the production of urine and to prevent spasms. Also called sweet spirits of nitre, it was used on blisters.

The fact that several of Mr Boyle's receipts are included in the Physick Book suggests that he was a surgeon and or an apothecary.

To Make Lozenges for the Heart Burn

Take oysters' shells, well dried in an oven,
beat and sift them as fine as possible. With
half a pound of this powder, mix half a
pound of fine sugar beaten and sifted; wet
this with a spoonful or two of milk and
water to make in a very stiff paste, then
mould them into lozenges and bake them
in a cool oven. This does so effectively
sweeten that sour humour in the stomach
that caused this distemper, that it not only
prevents it but help digestion. To give you
a good opinion of this medicine, only try its
immediate power over the sharpest vinegar.

Mrs Vach's to make Rue Possett for Children that has Worms

Boil and handful or rue in a pint of milk
till it is pretty strong then put in a bit of
alum to turn it, but not too clear; strain
it and sweeten the whey with honey.
Give a quarter of a pint fasting and
the same quantity about five o'clock in
the afternoon.

Mrs Powell's Receipt for Cholick Water

Take of cloves, galangal, cubebs, mace,
lesser cardamoms, nutmeg, ginger of each
half an ounce, of French brandy, five full
quarts. Pound the ingredients and let
them lie in the brandy two days, close covered, then distil it in a cold still, adding
three pints of water.
If it be done in an alembic, there must be
a gallon of water put to it and five quarts
drawn off with a moderate fire. When it
is distilled, put it into a glass jar and put
to it two ounces of the best rhubarb sliced
and let it infuse two or three days, then
strain it off and bottle it.

Pint: the British imperial pint was not introduced until the nineteenth century, so the pint mentioned in Elizabeth Ambler's Physick Book was equivalent to 16 fluid ounces, as is the American one.

Colic: also written 'cholic', 'cholick' and 'colick', is abdominal pain and cramp. Renal colic can be caused by kidney disease and affects the ureter. Gallstone colic is caused by stones in the bile duct. Strictly speaking, it refers to the colon but is generally applied to any disorder of the stomach or bowels that causes pain, and is also referred to as the gripes and bellyache. Johnson wrote: 'Strictly a disorder of the colon but loosely any disorder of the stomach or bowels that is attended with pain, also gripes and bellyache.'

Cubebs: the fruit of the *Piper cubeba*, which is also known as the cubeb pepper. A native of Java, it is related to cardamom and has a very strong taste which some liken to allspice, while others describe it as being more like eucalyptus.

Mrs Berry's Receipt for syrup of marsh mallows which is a fine cooling opening slippery syrup and chiefly commendable for the Cholick in the kidneys or bladder or the Gravel

Take of marshmallows roots two ounces, red cicers an ounce, of the roots of grass asparagus and liquorish, raisins of the sun stoned, of each half an ounce, the branches of marshmallows, pellitory of the wall, burnet, plantain, maiden hair, fern both white and black of each a handful, of the four greatest and the four lesser cold seeds, of each three drams. Boil them in six pints of water until only four remain to which add four pounds of sugar and boil it to a syrup. Be sure you boil it enough, for if you boil it never so little too little it will quickly sour.

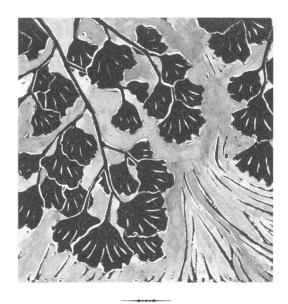

Cicers: *Cicer arietinum*, better known as chickpeas, were used to induce menstruation, produce urine and help in the treating of kidney stones.

Pellitory of the wall: *Parietaria diffusa*, known to be good for stone and urinary problems.

Cold seeds: probably those of pumpkins or their near relations, traditionally effective in getting rid of intestinal worms.

Mr Walder's Receipt for the Tincture for Gout and Colick in Stomach

2½ pounds of raisins, chopped
½ pound of rhubarb, shred very thin
2 ounces senna
1 ounce coriander seeds
1 ounce fennel seeds
1 ounce cochineal
½ ounce of saffron
½ ounce of liquorish

Infuse these in two gallons of best brandy;
let it stand 10 days in a large bottle,
sometimes stirring it, then strain it off and
put in five quarts of brandy. Let it remain
for a month or six weeks; it will be as good
as the first.
Take a wine glass when the pain is troublesome and if the pain is not better in
two hours, take another.
The quarter of this quantity is enough
to make at a time.

Gout: a very painful disease characterised by inflammation of the smaller joints, typically those in the toe, caused by an excess of uric acid salts in the blood of the sufferer. Sufferers are usually portrayed humorously, and unsympathetically, as fat, elderly men nursing a big toe which is encased in yards of bandages, but the truth is that gout can occur in several parts of the body, including the heel, knee, wrist and finger as well as cause the formation of stones. The reason that gout was so common in the eighteenth century is the high consumption of red meat and fortified wines. It was sometimes referred to as the rich man's disease.

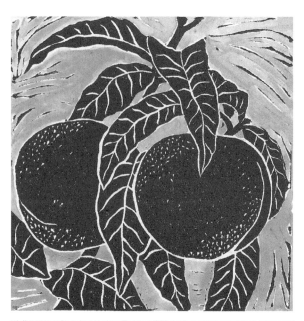

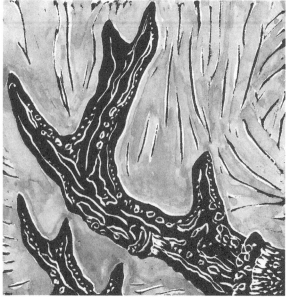

A high Cordiall – water good against Surfeits and to Strengthen the Stomack our own way

Take 8 quarts of brandy and a peck of poppies, the black bottoms cutt away, and of cloves, gilly flowers, half a peck, the white bottoms cut away. Put them into brandy in a glass with a wide mouth and as will hold at least half a gallon more. Mint, balm, wood betony, sorrell, hyssop, pennyroyal, and all together alike, a handfull of each; marigold flowers half a handfull, a little agrimony, black cherrys, 3 pound of figs, ½ a pound raisins of the sun, stoned, ½ a pound blue currants, ½ a pound sweet fennill seeds, caraways and aniseeds plucked and bruised, of each an ounce, liquorish scraped and still too thin, and sugar, 1 pound. Stir it once a day and let it stand a fortnight, then bottle it up. The dose is for a man, a quart, for a woman, 3 quarters of the quart, for youths half the quart.

Surfeit water: a medicinal drink designed to cure over-indulgence in eating and drinking.

Lady Piles's Receipt for a Wind Cholick or any Cholicks, which gives ease soon if they are violent

To a quart of brandy put one ounce of Virginia snake root and half an ounce of cochineal; two or three spoonfuls is a dose to drink.

If the cholick is very bad and there is no evacuation, the following glisters —

A quarter of a pint of sack or good mountain wine, half a pint of the decoction of camomile flowers, the yolk of a new-laid egg. Beat the egg and the wine together, [with] two ounces of brown sugar; mix all these together and strain it then add 15 drops oil of caraway, four spoonfuls salat oil. If you would have it more purging add two or three spoonfuls of syrup of violets.

The quieting glister: Two hours after, if the pain continues, 50 drops of laudanum in four spoonfuls of chicken's water to be taken as a glister and repeated in two hours if the pain continues, adding 10 drops more of laudanum. Should you not be quite eased, begin again with the first glister.

Glister: also spelt 'clyster', is an old word for an enema.

Mountain wine: any fortified wine from Malaga, which was grown in the mountains immediately to the north of that town.

Sack: see note on P. 55.

Mrs Cottenham's Receipt to make Bitters for the Wind Cholick

Take a quart of raisin wine, put to it three quarters of an ounce of the best bark powdered, two drams of snakeroot, one dram of saffron, one dram of cochineal, bruised, the yellow rind of six Seville oranges. When it has stood 84 hours, strain it off and fill the bottle of ingredients again, which you may do three times and it will be good. Drink a wineglass of it an hour before dinner and at 5 or 6 o'clock in the afternoon if the patient is costive, slice a bit of rhubarb in the ingredients.

Costive: constipated.

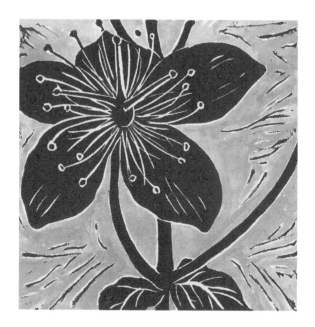

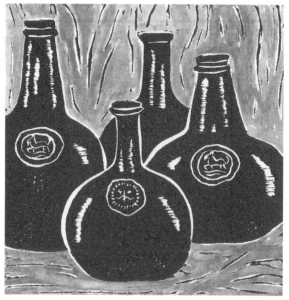

Respiratory

Receipt for Whooping Cough in Children

Take dried coltsfoot leaves, a good handful, cut them small and boil them in a pint of spring water till half a pint is boiled away. Then take it off the fire and when almost cold strain it through a cloth, squeezing the herb as dry as you can and dissolve in the liquor an ounce of brown sugar candy finely powdered and then give the child one spoonful of it, cool or warm as the season proves, 3 or 4 times a day or oftener if the fits prove frequently. It is very good for all sorts of coughs in young or old, shortness of breath and all other things incident to coughs and colds.

Mrs Coppinger's Receipt for Plaster to a Child's Stomach that has a Shortness of Breath and a Cough

Take one ounce of Venice Treacle, one ounce of strained Burgundy Pitch, one ounce of rosin, one ounce of beeswax; put them all into a pan and when 'tis dissolved on a gentle fire, let it stand a little and scum off the dross and pour the clear from the settlement into an other pan, and add one ounce of oil of mace and one ounce of oil of nutmeg. When they are well incorporated together put them into a gallipot. It must be the chimical oil of nutmeg and the pressed oil of mace.

Burgundy pitch: the sap of a spruce tree found in alpine valleys and still collected for use as incense and for its antibacterial properties.

Rosin: resin, also spelled rossom.

Mace: the dried outer covering of the nutmeg. One of its main uses today is as one of the spices in Christmas puddings.

Gallipot: A small, glazed earthenware jar used by druggists for holding medicaments such as ointment or tablets.

Chimical oil: volatile or essential oil.

Mr Knape's Receipt for the Hooping Cough

Shave of the hair of the head the bigness of ½ a crown. Dip a piece of {fools} cap brown paper in oil of amber; as it dries wet it, it cures 2 or 3 times.

This refers, of course, to whooping cough, so called because of the sound that the sufferer makes. It was also called 'chin cough', a name which is still found in some dialects today.

Mrs Rushton's Receipt for a Cough

Sugar candy beat to powder	2 oz
Candied Eli compane beat to powder	2 oz
Conserve of red roses	1 oz
Conserve of rosemary blossoms	1 oz
Oil of sweet almonds	1 oz

Syrup of maidenhair, as much as is sufficient to make it into a consistence for a bolus.

Take the quantity of a large nutmeg when the cough is troublesome, for a grown person and the quantity of a little nutmeg for a child.

Eli compane: (elecampane) *Inula helenium*, a plant which resembles the sunflower and has bitter aromatic leaves which were used in both medicine and cookery. Its root was used to treat scabies and the itch as well as coughs, snake bites, convulsions and bruising. It is an important medicinal root.

Maidenhair: *Adiantum capillus-veneris* is a type of fern used to lessen congestion in the lungs and treat coughs, bronchitis, whooping cough and heavy menstruation with abdominal cramps.

Women's Health

Mrs Cartwright's Receipt to Stop a Flooding

Take a pint of red wine and put in a handful of blackberries' buds and boil it up till it is very strong and take a cupful of it every night and morning; sweeten it with treble-refine sugar to your taste.

Flooding: abnormally heavy bleeding during menstruation.

Mrs Freeman's Receipt to Stop Flooding

Burn a piece of new Holland that has never been washed, to tinder then powder it and mix a tea-spoonful of it in a large spoon with red wine and take it night and morning and drink a little red wine after it.

Holland: a cloth named after its country of origin. It was initially a fine brownish-coloured plain linen fabric.

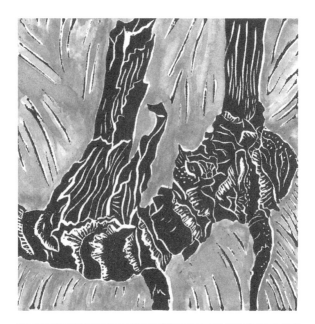

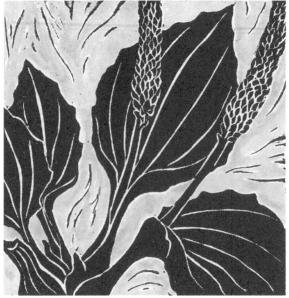

Dr Nisbitt's Receipt for a Flooding

Take a chicken, skin and bone it, or a
pound of mutton without fat or bone, put
it into a quart of cold water and boil it up
but once, keeping it skimmed at the time
it is boiling. Then take the meat out and
cut it into pieces, then put it into the same
water it boiled in, then boil it altogether
just six minutes. Then strain it off and let
the patient drink often on it. They must
drink a quarter of a pint at a time. It will
increase their blood as fast as they lose it
and recover them from fainting.

Mrs Lawrance's Receipt to Prevent a Miscarriage or to Strengthen Anybody after it Happens

Take twelve knuckles or shank bones or legs or shoulders of mutton; put them in a pan of water for two or three hours. Rub them with a little salt and wash them very clean. Put in to a pot with a gallon of spring water, let it boil an hour and scum it very clean, then put in two ounces of hartshorn shavings and the bottom of a halfpenny roll. Let it boil till it comes to about 3 pints then strain it off. When cold, take off the fat.

Take half a pint as warm as you can about an hour before you rise, and the same quantity going to bed. This receipt is an approved one.

Mrs Lane's Receipt for the Same Complaint

As the top written one: you must begin taking this jelly when first with child and continue till quick. 'Tis a great strengthener to drink after a miscarriage.

Take two ounces of hartshorn shavings and two ounces isinglass (of mace and cinnamon each ½ a dram); boil these in three pints of water till half is wasted, strain it off and sweeten it with white sugar candy.

N.B. take four spoonfuls of this jelly in a quarter of a pint of warm milk twice a day; if milk don't agree, it may be taken in red wine.

'These receipts meets with success.'

Isinglass: a type of gelatine obtained from the dried swim bladder of certain fish, notably the sturgeon but after 1795 a cheaper version was invented using cod. Isinglass is a type of collagen used to clarify wine and beer.

For a Weakness called the Whites

Take of white amber and mastic, finely
powdered, 3 drams, olibanum and fine
chalk in powder each one dram, of the
moss that grows upon oaken pales 2 scruples; make this into pills with as much
turpentine as will suffice.
Take the bigness of a white pea 3 times
a day, drinking after each a draught of
possett drink in which white comfrey has
been boiled with a little plantain: continue
this way until you have taken twice this
quantity, taking a little rhubarb with
grated nutmeg once in three days. Pray
to take the grated rhubarb and nutmeg at
night, going to bed.

The Whites: leucorrhoea, a whitish yellow or greenish vaginal discharge which indicates inflammation or congestion of the mucous membranes of the vagina or the uterus. It is interesting that all of the remedies in Elizabeth's book for this complaint feature white ingredients, in this one white amber, chalk and white pea and in others oatmeal and parsnip.

Mastic: the resin of the mastic tree, *Pistacia lentiscus*. It starts off as a liquid which is then dried in the sun to form drops of hard, brittle, translucent resin. The idea that mastic is useful for alleviating colds and digestive disorders goes back to Hippocrates.

Olibanum: frankincense.

Possett: a drink made of hot milk curdled with ale, wine or other alcohol and often spiced. It was popular from medieval to Victorian times and given to sufferers of colds and similar indispositions as a comfort drink. Nowadays the word is used to refer to a type of pudding.

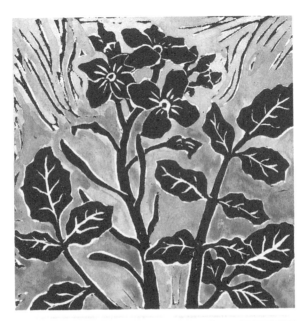

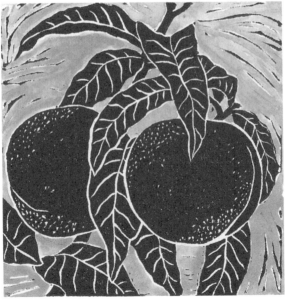

Aches and Pains

Mr Boyle's Receipt for Chilblains

Take thick, fresh parings of turnips
and hold them to the fire till they be
crisp, then apply them to the unbroken
tumours or blisters, as hot as the patient
can endure.
Keep them on for a competent time and
apply new if need require. They will cause
the peccant to transpire or otherwise
waste, without breaking the blisters.

Peccant: the cause of the condition.

Tobacco for the Eyes

Take the best plain tobacco, 4 ounces
betony, 3 handfuls coltsfoot, the flowers of
rosemary and lavender of each two handfuls, storax and amber, of each an ounce.
Let the storax and amber be pulverised
then mix them all well together, use.

Mrs Parish's Receipt to Strengthen Hands that have been Broke

Take the yolk of an egg and throw a
spoonfull of water on it and beat it
together, then throw another spoonfull of
water on it again then beat it up together
and then throw the third spoonfull
of water and beat it again and let the
patient wash their hands with it two or
three times a day; it has recovered several
people's strength after such an accident.

To Cure a Pain of the Head which Returns at Sett Times like an Ague

Take 2 scruples of Jesuits' Bark, make it into a bolas with a sufficient quantity of syrup of gillyflowers, to be repeated every six hours being constantly taken for three days; it seldom fails of success.

Jesuits' Bark: or Peruvian bark, comes from the cinchona tree, which is dried and powdered. It contains quinine which is used against malaria; this was still prevalent in Britain in Elizabeth's day. The word 'Jesuit' refers to the part that this religious order played in the colonisation of Latin America.

Gillyflowers: any of a number of sweet-smelling flowers including the wallflower or white stock; formerly a clove-scented pink or carnation.

Bolas: a large pill; via the Latin from the Greek *bōlos* 'clod', it is generally used today in veterinary medicine.

Mrs Ambler's Receipt for a Hoarseness

Take of decoction of senna, three ounces,
of syrup of buckthorn one ounce, of
compound of peony water half an ounce,
make it a purging potion to be taken early
in the morning. Two or three takes after
the taking of the purge, draw ten ounces
of blood from the arm. Take of the gum
ammoniac a dram, hog-lice prepared, one
dram and a half, of liquorish juice, balsam
of Tolu, spermaceti, of each half a dram,
syrup of maidenhair a sufficient quantity.
Make 'em into sixty middle-sized pills,
and four to be taken every morning and
evening in one spoonful of the mixture;
drinking four spoonfuls of the julep
underneath mentioned.
Take of the syrup of maidenhair and of the
juice of ground ivy of each an ounce and a
half, of the tincture of saffron one ounce,
make nit into a mixture.
Take of milk water eight ounces, of compound peony water two ounces and a half,
syrup of balsam, one ounce: make it into
a julep.

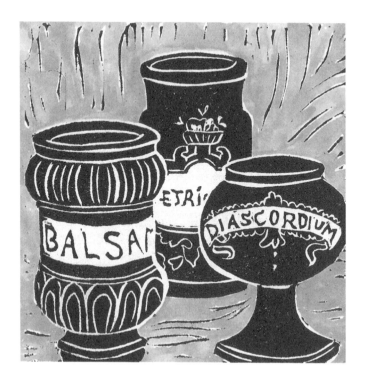

Senna: the seeds of the cassia shrub, which are used as an emetic and a laxative.

Hog-lice: this is more likely to refer to woodlice which have other pig-related names, and appear in other receipts rather than the true hog-lice which live on swine.

Nurse Payne's Receipt for a Sore Throat in the Small Pox

Take honey to the quantity of two large spoonfulls, as thick as you can get it, rock allum, burnt enough to cover a sixpence or a shilling, a little surrup of mulberries to colour them and as much dog's white turd as will lay upon a sixpence, finely pounded, and take a little in a teaspoon as you shall find occasion.

Rock alum: alum, or aluminum sulfate, occurs in nature as the mineral alunogenite. It is used as an astringent, a styptic and an emetic, but is dangerous in the wrong hands as it is an irritant and corrosive; swallowing as little as 30g (1oz) has killed adults. Between the mid-seventeenth and mid-nineteenth century, Ravenscar, a village between Whitby and Scarborough in Yorkshire, was one of the world's leading producers of alum. This substance, which was produced from local shale, was used to cure leather and as a fixative for dyes, as well as in medicine. Alum was extracted by means of huge bonfires which were kept alight for months, after which human urine (collected from all over the country and imported by the boatload) was poured over the heaps of rock.

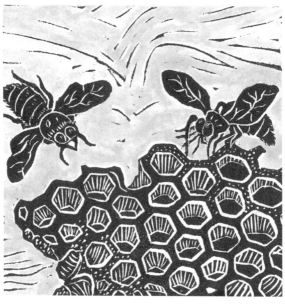

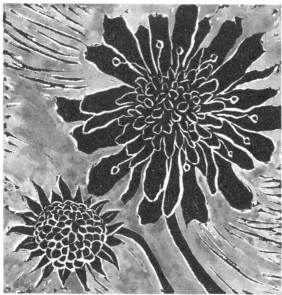

For the Tooth Acke

Take the root of pelitory of Spain, dip'd
seven times in mountain wine as often as
dry dip it again. Apply a bit to the tooth
afflicted, it will preserve and
give ease.

Root of pelitory of Spain: this refers to a composite
plant, *Anacyclus pyrethrum*, with a pungent root
which is still used as a local irritant; it relieves
toothache by causing the patient to salivate
freely. A tincture made from the dried root and
rubbed on to the gum or put on to cotton wool
will relieve aching teeth. Reports of its efficiency
as a proven remedy survive from thirteenth-
century Wales, and pelitory remains a favourite
today in Eastern countries.

Mrs Goodchild's Receipt for the Tooth Acke

Pelitory of Spain, gum ammoniac, grains of paradise, an equal quantity of all the ingredients bruised small, and lay some of it to the tooth that aches.

Gum ammoniac: the hardened juice of an umbelliferous plant, *Dorema ammoniacum*, used to treat bronchial problems. It is closely related to asafoetida. It is now used in gilding.

Paradise: *Aframomum melegueta* is a member of the ginger family.

Mrs Grinly's Receipt a Certain Cure for the Tooth Acke

Take a bit of lint and put a bit of Norway tar upon it and put it to your tooth; it will make you a little sick, but it will relieve the pain.

Norway tar: a brown, liquid tar thought by some to be the best to use when making tar-water, which was made by mixing the tar with cold water, storing and bottling it. It was recommended for the 'curing of most diseases, particularly all foul cases, ulcers and eruptions, scurvies of all kinds, nervous disorders, inflammatory distempers, decays, etc.' (Taken from a letter by the author of *Siris*, in the *Dublin Journal*, 8–12 May 1724).

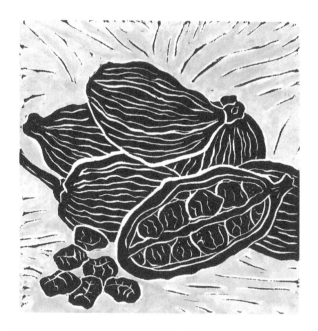

Mr Perrot's Receipt for the Tooth Acke

Horseradish, mustard, cinnamon, white wine vinegar, mix them together and let them simmer some time over the fire, then snuff the liquor up your nose on the opposite side from where the pain is and continue it until the pan is gone; hold your pulse on the opposite side from the pain. It will operate 'by way of sallavating [salivating]'.

A Receipt for Lip Salve Mrs Willis's Way

Take two-pennyworth of Alcona root,
steep it in 6 spoonfulls of sweet oyl; lett
it stand all night then strain it. Put to
it 9 pennyworth of white virgins wax,
6 pennyworth of natureall balsam; let it
symmer over the fire in a pipkin till all be
melted then pour it into the bottom of
cups, wetting them.

Alcona root: probably alkanet, *Alkanna tinctoria* (also known as *Anchusa tinctoria*), a relation of borage. The inner part of the root of the plant gives a reddish-purple colorant which is added to oils and spirits of wine as well as for dyeing. French ladies were reported to paint their faces with this root.

Receipt for the Rheumatism

An ounce of winter bark bruised, and
ounce of horseradish root sliced or scraped,
a large handful of scurvy grass bruised,
2 spoonfuls of mustard seed bruised. Put
them into a large bottle and pour a quart
of mountain wine on them. Let it stand
twelve hours stopped close and then take
three wineglassfuls every day; one of the
glasses should be taken [when] going to
rest and wrapped warm. After the first
3 glasses are taken out, every time after
that you take one out, put one in of fresh
wine to the quantity of a pint more.
Strain it through a piece of muslin or it
will be foul and disagreeable to drink
and a small glass of about 3 spoonfuls is
enough for women.

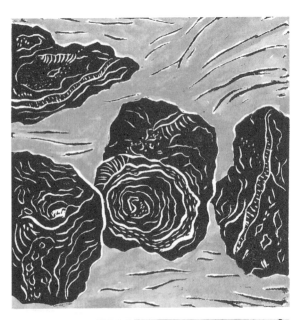

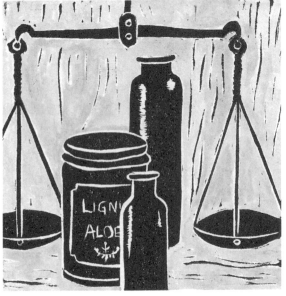

Assorted Maladies

<u>Mrs Cleeves's Receipt for Convulsion Fitts</u>

Take the herb lady's smock, the sort which looks of a pale blush, the colour just turned from the white, which is generally found in meadows the beginning of April and distil them in a cold still. Dry some flowers and young leaves together to powder; sift it through a fine sieve and give to a young child as much as will lie on a threepence in a spoonful of the distilled water two or three times a day if the fit be upon it, or else only in the morning three days before the full moon and three days or so before and after the change of the moon. If the child be a year old, give as much as will be on a sixpence and to a grown person as such as to be on a shilling or more. If you have not the distilled water of the same herb, honey water or black cherry water is very good. To dry the flowers in a chamber without fire or sun is the best way.

An Often Experienced Remedy to Expel Gravel and Provoke Supprest Urine

Take the thick membrane that lines the
gizzard of a cock or hen and having wip'd
it clean, dry it so that it may be beaten to
powder. With this mix an equal part of
choice red coral calcinat'd and of the mixture give from 20 or 30 to 40 or 50 grains.

Gravel: a disease in which small stones formed in
the kidneys, pass along the ureter to the bladder, and are expelled in the urine. Johnson
defined it as 'Sandy matter concreted in the kidneys'. Today it is called a stone in the kidneys.
Calcinated: roasted or burnt.

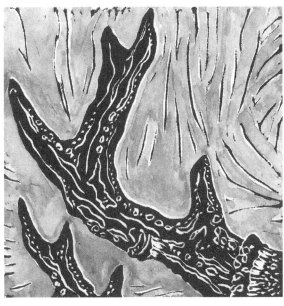

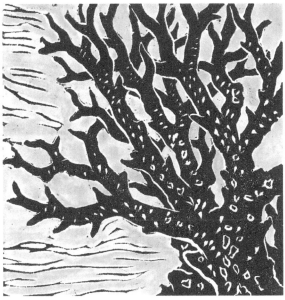

Mr Perkins's Receipt for the Stone Dissolving it and Bringing it Away

Take six lemons, cut them in the middle and squeeze them into an earthen cup and strain them twice through a cloth and put six spoonfuls of powder[ed] fine white sugar candy into it and six spoonfuls of the very best salat oil and scrape a small bit of Castile soap into it, as big as the top of your little finger and stir it all very well together and drink it all off at once, in the morning fasting and fast 3 or 4 hours after the taking of it.

Ironically, Elizabeth's own son, Elisha Biscoe, was to die from an operation to remove a bladder stone, doubtless after trying all the medical alternatives available to him at the time. His niece, Letitia, wrote:

My Uncle, having suffered for some time, not so much from actual pain as inconvenience and mental Feelings from the progressive growth of a stone in the bladder, departed this life on

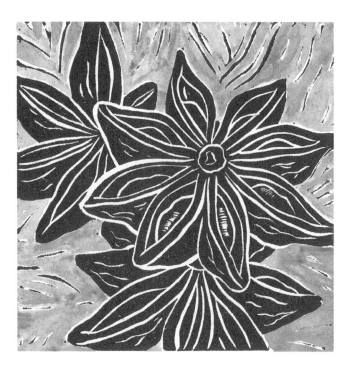

the 10th of April 1829, the actual cause of his
decease being from a trial by Mr Henry Earle
of breaking the stone, which proved abortive
and brought on the Fatal catastrophe.

Henry Earle was a noted and well-respected surgeon; he was related to the Biscoe family through
the marriage of Elizabeth's daughter Anne to
Timothy Earle of Swallowfield.

Mrs Whitefield's Receipt for Green Sickness

Conserve of Roman wormwood, of red roses, of borage flowers each one ounce, prepared steel two drams, powder of cinnamon two scruples, preserved citrus peel two drams and a half, salt of wormwood two scruples, saffron eight grains, syrup of citrus peel a sufficient quantity to make it into an electuary.

Take the quantity of a nutmeg in the morning fasting, and drink a glass of white wine afterwards, if you please it should be taken again in the afternoon and fast two hours after some time. If better, you can omit it in the afternoon; use moderate exercise.

Conserve: a type of jam in which the fruit is left whole or in large pieces.

Green sickness: chlorosis, a chronic form of anaemia usually of girls around the age of puberty, caused by an iron and protein deficiency, which gives a greenish-yellow tinge to the skin. It was known as virgin's pallor or virgin's disease and is mentioned several times by Shakespeare.

Mrs Simmon's Receipt for Jaundice

Take a large lemon, cut off the top, and put into it a dram of saffron and a little cochineal and put it into the lemon, then put it into a saucer to roast as you do an apple. Then slice it into a basin and get a pint of the best mountain [wine] and simmer it and pour on it and cover your basin all night. And take it in a morning fasting, a teacupful a little warm, and another at going to bed. 'Tis best to take a vomit first and then a little powder of rhubarb, and now and then leaving off the medicine the days you take the rhubarb, smoking a pipe of tobacco in the morning. Fasting is very good with this medicine, and keep to the above rules till you find yourself cured.

Jaundice: Dr Johnson defined this as 'a distemper from obstruction of the glands of the liver which prevents the gall from being duly separated from the blood'.

Mr Nicolls Receipt to Make Aqua Paralytica or Palsy Water

Take of lavender flowers stript from their stalks and fill with them a large gallon glass and pour on them of the best spirits of wine as much as will cover them. Macerate them for six weeks, being close stopt and clad with a bladder so that nothing may breathe out and let them stand in a warm place, then distil them in a limbeck {alembic} with his cooler, then put into the said water, flowers of sage, rosemary {and} betony, of each an handful and of flowers of borage, bugloss, cowslips, lily of the valley, of each one handful. Steep the flowers in good Malmsey or spirits of wine, every one in his season, till all may be had. Put to them also, balm, motherwort spike flowers, bay leaves, the leaves of orange trees and their flowers, of each one ounce. Cut all small and put into the aforesaid distilled wine and distil them as before, being steeped six weeks, and when it is distilled put into it citron piece and peony seeds hulled, of each, six drams, cinnamon half an ounce,

nutmegs, mace, cardamoms, cubebs,
yellow saunders, of each one ounce, and
lignum aloes, one dram. Make all of these
into fine powder, put them into the above
said distilled water and put to them of
jujubes, new and good, half a pound (first
stoned before you weigh them) cut small
then close your vessel with a double bladder. Let them digest six weeks then strain
these with a press and filtrate the liquor,
then put therein prepared pearl two
drams, smeradgus prepared one scruple,
ambergris, musk, saffron of each half a
scruple, red roses well dried {and} sweet
smelling red and yellow saunders of each
one ounce. Hang all these in a sarsnet
bag in the water, well close that nothing
breathe out – the intention of this medica-
ment is against the falling sickness and all
cold distempers of the head, womb, stomach and nerves as {well as}the apoplexy,
palsy, convulsions, megrim, vertigo, loss of
memory, dimness of sight, swooning fits
and barrenness in women. You may give
to a child from a scruple to a dram, to a
man one dram to four.
It is an excellent by {but} costly medicine.

Palsy: paralysis especially when accompanied by involuntary tremors; the best-known types are Bell's and cerebral palsies. Parkinson's disease is sometimes called shaking palsy. Dr Johnson's definition is: 'a privation of motion or feeling or both, proceeding from some cause below the cerebellum, joined with a coldness, flaccidity, and at last wasting of the parts. If affecting all the parts below the head, except the thorax and heart it is called a paraplegia, if in one side only a hemiplegia; if in some parts only on one side, a paralysis.'

Bladder: a sheep's or ox's bladder used to make an airtight covering.

Macerate: to soften by placing in a liquid.

Motherwort: *Leonurus cardiaca*, prescribed for the prevention of uterine infection; it is also good for the heart and promoting general relaxation.

Musk: a substance with a distinctive and strong scent. It is secreted by a gland common to several animals, notably the musk deer.

Saunders: also called sandalwood, is the tree *Santalum album* which is native to India. In medieval times its wood was made into a compound used as a dark-red food colouring. Red saunders or sanders, also called red sandalwood or rubywood, comes from the tree *Pterocarpus santalinus*, also found in the Subcontinent. Apart from its medicinal use as an astringent and tonic, it was used for dyeing and in cosmetics. It should not be confused with the true sandalwood, *Santalum album*. Saunders is also a corruption of the name of the umbelliferous vegetable, alexanders.

Lignum aloes: the resinous wood of *Aquilaria agallocha*, a large tree which is grown in Malaysia. Known in English as aloe wood or eagle wood, until recently it was used as incense.

Jujubes: *Ziziphus zizyphus*, also known as red date, Chinese date, Korean date or Indian date, is soothing for the throat and claimed to relief stress; it is antibacterial.

Smeradgus: an old name for emerald.

Sarsnet or sarsenet: very fine and soft silk material.

Falling sickness: epilepsy.

Apoplexy: paralysis caused by stroke. Johnson's definition is: 'Sudden deprivation of all the internal and external sensation and of all motion unless of the heart and thorax.'

Megrim: in this context it means migraine, but is also a kind of fish.

Conclusion

In his Receipt against Plague, Sir Walter Raleigh wrote: 'Keep this as your life above all worldly treasures.' This demonstrates the importance of these remedies; people depended on them just as we rely on antibiotics and medicine today. We are fortunate now to have much more protection from disease and ill health. Elizabeth and her family had good reason to treasure her Physick Book: many of the cures and remedies would have been extremely effective and many used on a regular basis.

It would be tempting to try making such remedies as Viper Broth and Snail Milk Water. It would also be intriguing to taste Venice Treacle or Balsam of Peru, and to sample more complex receipts containing ingredients such as ambergris, red coral, pearls and emeralds. However, we should be cautious about trying any of the receipts ourselves; many of the ingredients contain powerful chemicals and experimentation would be extremely dangerous. We can appreciate and marvel at the multitude of ingredients – plants, animals and minerals – but must leave it to the pharmacologists to investigate and refine them for use in medicinal preparations. There is still a great need for discoveries in this field and we will certainly need them in the future. I know that both my aunts, Diana and Dorothy, would have been glad to see the 'old recipe book' being shared and appreciated more widely. I expect Elizabeth herself – and also Anne, Letitia and Fanny – would be rather surprised to see the publication of familiar family receipts, but I hope they would also be pleased. I am grateful to them for passing the book down through the family. Not only have I found my discoveries about their lives so interesting and inspiring, but I also feel I have gained a strong sense of continuity and connection with the past.

Nicola Lillie
2013

About the Authors

Marilyn Yurdan attended Holton Park Grammar School for Girls in Oxfordshire during the 1950s. She went on to work as Assistant Custodian at the University of Oxford's Sheldonian Theatre for twenty-two years. She has been awarded a Master of Studies in English Local History from the University of Oxford, and has written numerous books, including *Oxford in the 1950s and '60s*.

Nicola Lillie is a descendant of Elizabeth Ambler and owner of the book of cures. She is an artist, producing murals and sculpted reliefs for interiors, and has taught Art at Oxford Brookes University.

Illustrator *Laura Lillie* has a First Class Honours degree and an MA with Distinction in Fine Art Printmaking.